I0458905

Turning on the Light

Kirk House Publishers

To Lily and Alena

TURNING ON

the

LIGHT

My Mysterious Illness and the Year that Transformed Me

SUSAN BRUZAS

Turning on the Light: My Mysterious Illness and the Year that Transformed Me Copyright © 2025 Susan Bruzas

All rights reserved. No part of this book may be used or reproduced in any manner whatsoever without written permission of the author, except in the case of brief quotations embodied in critical articles and reviews.

First printing, August 2025
First edition

Paperback ISBN: 978-1-959681-88-5
eBook ISBN: 978-1-959681-90-8
Hardcover ISBN: 978-1-959681-89-2

Library of Congress Control Number: 2025912176

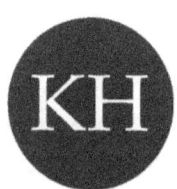

Published by Kirk House Publishers
1250 E 115th Street
Burnsville, MN 55337
612-781-2815
To order, visit: kirkhousepublishers.com
Quantity discounts are available.

TABLE OF CONTENTS

Chapter 1

AN ICY TOUCH

It was a warm July afternoon in 2015. The shades were drawn in my bedroom, and candlelight shone on the walls. The steady thrum of an Indian tamboura was playing on a CD. I silently repeated the mantra given to me by my guru—one repetition on the in-breath, and another on the out-breath until eventually I dropped into a serene, loving, and very familiar space within myself.

Icy fingers touched my wrist. I gasped, and my whole body jerked. I was ripped out of meditation. My eyes flew open, and I looked around. Nothing was there. No one was anywhere near me. I lived alone with my cat, William, who was outside on the deck sleeping. William has no fingers.

I took several deep breaths to try to calm myself. This wasn't the first time this summer that these wintry fingers had touched me. It always seemed to happen during meditation. How many times had it been? Two? Three? More importantly, what could it be? The touch didn't feel malevolent. Was this someone I knew who had died? What did this entity want? My attention? On what? Did it want to take me with it?

A chill went down my spine, and I pulled the shawl around me. Many times, after someone close to me had died, I would have an experience of that person.

Once years before, when I was in the stage between sleep and wakefulness, I sensed my mother and her sister standing at the end of my bed, both of them looking at me. "Oh, she's okay," my mom whispered to my aunt. Then they turned away, clasped each other's hands, and skipped off quite happily. They seemed young and carefree. I was reassured to see that my mom was with the one person she'd been closest to in her long life.

This icy touch did *not* feel like my mother.

Was it my *dad's* mother? Granny's life had been difficult. She'd been abandoned at thirteen by a father and stepmother who didn't want her or her nine-year-old brother. Her father had finally arranged for her to marry a man in his twenties. That was my grandfather. The marriage had been tumultuous, but Granny raised four kids and managed a beauty school in Seattle. I was proud of her.

One night a few months after her death, she'd appeared to me in a dream. I saw my grandmother, standing alone before me, wearing a long black dress.

She told me, "I want to meet your guru."

I was surprised. I'd never mentioned my guru or anything about meditation to my grandmother. I didn't think she'd understand.

I asked her, "You want to meet my guru?"

"I've got to try something."

She sounded desolate. I took her by the hand. It was ice cold.

In the dream, the two of us walked over to my guru, who seemed to be waiting for us. My guru was wearing the traditional orange robes of an Indian monk. It's what she usually wears. I stood beside her and took hold of my grandmother's cold, cold hand. Pulling my granny with me, I melted into my beloved teacher. My guru became a huge, bright flame. Granny and I were both enveloped by love.

I had never dreamed of my grandmother again. Was this her now? Was she trying to warn me about something?

Recently, during meditation I had seen my framed print of Goddess Lakshmi—the deity of wealth and well-being—fall from its place on top of my wardrobe. This had happened several times. Each time, I put my arm out, trying to stop the picture from falling to the floor. But when I opened my eyes, Lakshmi would be in her rightful place, on top of the wardrobe, unharmed.

It occurred to me: maybe I should tell someone about all of this.

♦   ♦   ♦

"I think there is an earthquake coming, and you'd better get prepared!" I told my friends.

We were at the meditation center, sitting around one of the circular tables in the community room. We'd just finished the early morning chant we did every Sunday. The doors were open to let in a cool morning breeze on what promised to be another hot summer day. I was enjoying a cup of hot chai and a warm, freshly baked blueberry scone.

"Do you mean the big one?" one woman asked me. She was referring to the number ten earthquake that has long been predicted for the Seattle area.

"Yes, I think so."

"Really?" My friend Mary Lou Finley looked at me intently with enigmatic blue eyes. "Why do you think that?"

Mary Lou and I had met at the meditation center thirty years ago. We both had daughters too young to be chanting and meditating with the adults, so the two of us chose to sit in the community room and entertain our children. The kids had become best friends, and so had we.

"For several weeks now, I've had visions of my Lakshmi picture falling," I said in a quiet voice. "Since Lakshmi is the goddess of good fortune, I'm thinking that maybe her falling means *bad* fortune! At first, I was afraid I'd done something like make a big mistake with my finances. But what if it's a calamity that will happen to us all? Like an earthquake. . ."

I talked on. The others at the table finished their breakfasts and drifted away. Mary Lou stayed and listened intently to me. Finally, she put a really positive spin on it. She said, "You always have amazing meditation experiences, Susan."

"I would just as soon not have this one over and over again. It's unnerving."

I decided not to tell her about the icy touch. I didn't want to freak her out.

"I can't remember," Mary Lou said, "but have you ever had visions that have come true?"

I took a breath in. "Well, I used to have dreams that a storm was approaching, and I would be terrified that something awful was about to happen. I had one where I was standing in my dining room looking out over the backyard. All of the leaves on the trees were spinning around wildly in the wind. I thought, 'This is going to be the worst storm I've ever seen.' And you know what happened?"

"What?"

"My brother was diagnosed with stage-three melanoma, my niece was severely hurt in a car accident, and her nine-year-old daughter was killed."

"Oh my God."

"Yep. And it didn't stop with that. A little while later my mom died."

"That's incredible, Susan."

"The Lakshmi photo falling wasn't a dream. It was a vision. And it definitely could be a warning."

Later, I went home and checked my earthquake readiness kit to make sure my emergency bottles of water were intact and that I had a can opener stored with my cans of food. All was well. I moved my Lakshmi picture off the top of my wardrobe and onto a small table in the living room. Maybe that would stop the visions of her falling.

The visions of Lakshmi did stop, but other signs kept coming— and some of them were warnings from the physical universe.

For instance, later that summer, I was sitting at my computer answering emails. "How do you spell that?" I said aloud. I was so frustrated. "R-E-C-E-I-V-E?"

I couldn't seem to spell lately—or, anyway, I didn't have the confidence that I was spelling correctly. I looked up the word on my computer. I had been right. Again. I closed my eyes to type so I could finish my email. I checked the spelling, and all of the words seemed right. I tried closing my eyes some more, but my hands were shaking.

Why were my hands shaking? I tried holding my right hand with my left to type. It didn't work.

Was this just one more annoyance to add to the list of symptoms of old age? What was on the list now? Let's see: my left hand shaking badly, my running into the side of my garage with my car, a stabbing sensation on the left side of my head…

Maybe all of this was happening because I was exhausted all the time.

There was a knock on my front door. I went to the door and found my former tenant. She had just moved out of the downstairs studio I'd rented to her.

She seemed both apologetic and annoyed. She said, "Susan, the check is wrong."

I took the check from her and looked it over. "It says $150. Isn't that what I owe you?"

"Yes, that's correct, but when you wrote the number out, you said, 'One hundred dollars and fifty cents.'"

"Oh, my gosh. I'm so sorry." Embarrassed, I carefully wrote a new check.

This wasn't the only check that I had written incorrectly. I should really call my doctor!

Later that day, I began to meditate. I felt uneasy. What if I saw my Lakshmi picture falling again? But I was so tired that I started to drop into sleep instead of meditation. When a frigid hand grasped my wrist, I jumped.

"Ah-h-h!" I yelled. "Leave me alone!"

It *was* a warning. I can't say for sure from whom. But I was being warned to wake up, to pay attention to my fogginess… and my shaking hands… and my fatigue. I was being told to see my doctor and to get my labs done. I'd had lupus since I was thirteen. I'd been taking medications for it all that time. There were so many things that needed to be checked.

But I didn't heed the signs. Instead, I thought about remote forms of impending disaster. And I did nothing.

◆　◆　◆

The summer days passed, hot and lazy. Soon, it was the last day of July. It was Gurupurnima, a full moon day offered traditionally in India to gurus and meditation teachers. We were having a grand celebration at the meditation center that night. It was my favorite Indian holiday because it honored our gurus, and I loved my guru.

Before meeting my guru, I had looked desperately for a true, unchanging love, which I could never seem to find. Love slipped through my fingers like water. Then I'd met my teacher, and my life had truly begun to change. I started meditating every day and going to satsangs at the meditation center. An inner source of love was revealed that was always available. I just had to remember to access and hold onto it.

Before the satsang, I dressed carefully in a sky blue silk top and white pants. I put on my crystal neck *mala*—a string of sacred beads—that I'd bought while visiting India. I looked at my hair in the mirror.

If I could just cover up the bald spots better. Why was I getting them anyway? My mom would get them sometimes. That could be it.

Dropping my hairbrush in the sink, I grabbed my purse, went down the stairs to the garage, and got into my red Prius. As I drove down the block, a warm, scented breeze blew in my window. My neighbor Diane was in her yard, and I waved at her as I drove by.

It would be a long time before I saw my home and neighbors again.

♦   ♦   ♦

It was a wonderful satsang, but at the end I felt so weak that I had to hang onto a chair when we stood for the closing chant. I left early and made my way into the community room, where cake and ice cream were being served.

I sat down at an empty table with my cake, and soon Ann joined me. She was a quiet woman I'd gotten to know in a group studying ancient Indian scriptures. Ann and I started chatting about our desserts.

"Did you get the gluten or non-gluten cake?" I asked.

"Oh, I always get non-gluten," she said.

"I get the gluten. It always tastes moister to me."

"Gluten doesn't bother you?"

"Cookies chocolate seem sad Burger King," I said in a squeaky Mickey Mouse voice.

Ann's eyes widened.

I tittered feeling strangely detached from my body.

What? Was that me talking?

I tried once more.

"Picture cake gloating sugar."

Ann's frightened eyes grew larger. We both stood at once.

"Hospital!" I said.

"Yes, you're going to the hospital," she agreed. "You get your stuff, and I'll go get my car."

We dumped our cake, and she raced out the front door. I put on my sweater and sat on a bench to wait.

What the heck was happening to me?

I was feeling a bit numb and as if I were watching a movie. As people floated by, talking and laughing with each other, Mary Lou came into focus.

I thought maybe I should tell this very dear friend what was going on, but she looked distracted and, anyway, I was afraid my words would come out jumbled.

A few minutes later, I went outside and watched as Ann drove up in a light green Subaru. After I got into the car, Ann, who is a home care nurse, brought out a medical kit and took my blood pressure. I assumed it was to make sure I was okay to make the drive to the emergency room, but I didn't trust myself to formulate a question. It must have been all right because we started down the road.

It was the beginning of an odyssey that would transform my life forever.

Chapter 2

SOMETHING MUST
BE WRONG

The luminous full moon bathed everything in a silvery light and seemed to follow us protectively as we drove toward the hospital. I felt safe with Ann. Not only was she a home care nurse, she was experienced—she worked with patients all over Seattle. She was wearing such a pretty deep blue blouse. I looked down at my clothes. It seemed surreal that only little while ago I had put on this beautiful blue silk top and a crystal necklace *mala* that I wore only for special Indian celebrations. And now we were headed for the ER.

"So, your insurance plan covers Virginia Mason, right?" Ann asked, interrupting my thoughts.

"I think so. But they'd rather we went to Urgent Care instead of the hospital emergency room. I don't like Urgent Care—it's always jammed with people. Especially on a full moon night."

I bit my lip nervously. Was anything wrong with me? I was talking fine now. "Maybe I should call the consulting nurse and see what they say. They're always available."

I found the number on my phone. Having lupus for so many years made me cautious about always having emergency phone numbers and extra medications.

I quickly reached the nurse and put the phone on speaker so Ann could hear me describe my symptoms.

"Should we be driving to the hospital or Urgent Care?" I asked.

"Pull over right now and call 911. You could be having a stroke."

The world tipped dizzily for a moment. I looked at Ann with wide eyes. I thanked the nurse and rang off.

Ann said, "I'm glad traffic on Roosevelt is light tonight. It'll be easier to find a place to pull over."

A parking place seemed to appear magically. My hand was trembling so much that I gave the phone to Ann. She called 911 and told them what was happening. They said they would send the medics and needed to know where to meet us. Remembering the last three times they had come to my house for lupus related emergencies, I knew the fire department would come as well.

"What about the parking lot at Whole Foods? It's right up the road." Ann got the go ahead and hung up.

Time seemed to slow down as we drove the few miles to the store.

What was happening? This was frighteningly different from my lupus symptoms.

As we arrived at the parking lot the familiar sound of a siren pierced the quiet night. I always say a brief prayer when I hear a siren. But this time it was coming for me.

Soon brilliant flashing lights signaled the fire truck coming around the corner and into the lot. Although the night was warm, I shivered suddenly, crossed my arms tightly against my chest. I tried to remember to breathe.

"I'd better tell them where we are," Ann said. She opened the car door and got out. I leaned my head back against the seat and repeated my mantra.

A few minutes later, Ann got back into the car. "Well, they're cute," she said. We both burst out laughing. It felt so good to laugh.

Two firefighters came to the car carrying medical equipment.

A young and, indeed, handsome man smiled reassuringly as he opened my door. Shining a tiny flashlight in my eyes, he gently asked me questions.

"What's your name?"

"Susan Bruzas."

"How old are you?"

"Sixty-seven."

"Okay, follow the light."

As I looked side to side and around in circles, he asked me more standard questions. I seemed to do fine. He had me squeeze his hand and then raise my arms.

The other medic took my blood pressure and asked me more questions. I told him about the sharp pains in my head and having word-finding problems off and on during the past few weeks. I knew there were other symptoms, but I couldn't remember them at the time.

A few minutes later he said, "You're not having a stroke, but you'd better go to the emergency room. I'll call ahead so that they're ready for you."

As we drove to Virginia Mason, I told Ann, "It's a relief I'm not having a stroke."

"Yes, it is."

"Do you know your way?"

"Yeah, I had a doctor there."

For the rest of the trip, we were quiet.

◆　◆　◆

Once we pulled into the drop-off section of the hospital, a man seemed to be waiting for us. I was sure he would say there was no parking. Instead, he stood quietly while I got out of the car. Ann drove off to park the car. The man walked me in the door and to the check-in desk. I looked around, and there was no one else waiting. The assistant asked me for my insurance card, which I shakily fished from my wallet. She looked long at my face. Did she expect me to drop on the floor and have a seizure?

Then I was shown into a room and was surprised to see a cluster of nurses and a doctor. I was again questioned and tested. Then the nurse whisked me into a changing room. Ann arrived just as I was hurried away for a CAT scan.

Time began to pass in what felt like a slide show, first one scene etched in time, then another. Some of the slides were black, like a photo had been taken but there wasn't enough light to register an image. I remember nothing about the scan, how I got there, what it was like, or going back to my room to wait for the doctor.

After a while the doctor and a nurse came into the room. They looked very serious.

"Most of your test results came back normal," the doctor said. He looked down at the chart. "Your EKG showed a normal sinus rhythm, blood pressure was good, oxygenation. . ."

As he talked on, the nurse looked at me with concern.

Why was she looking at me that way? Something must be wrong.

Then I heard it: "…Unfortunately, your CT scan showed some edema in the left frontal lobe and the left temporal lobes, which are concerning for underlying masses."

I stared at him. The room and all its details seemed to disappear. There was just this pleasant-mannered doctor standing there, looking at me.

"Masses?"

His eyes softened. "Yes, the masses have metastasized and inflamed your brain in the speech area, and the pressure probably is what caused your jumbled talking."

"Did you say *metastasized*?"

He paused, glancing sideways at the nurse. "Yes, we will need to do an MRI, but given the two discrete areas affected, there is a concern for metastatic disease."

"Metastatic? You mean that I have cancer?"

He and the nurse nodded simultaneously.

"Cancer that has metastasized from somewhere else?"

"Most likely," the doctor said.

I was stunned into silence. Cancer? I had always thought that lupus was what would kill me. Cancer? It didn't make sense.

I looked at Ann. Horror flitted across her face. She was a nurse and knew from firsthand experience what I was facing. If there were metastasized tumors in my brain, they had been around for a while.

I forced myself to focus. I asked, "What's the plan for treatment?"

"We don't know as of yet. We're going to admit you and conduct more tests so that we can come up with a protocol of treatment."

♦ ♦ ♦

Eventually, they left. I settled down as comfortably as I could on the hard table. All was quiet except for the beeping of the cardiac monitor and buzzing of a light tube that needed changing. I looked at the clock. It was 2:00 a.m.

"Ann, you look tired. I'll be fine here. It's okay for you to go home."

"I'll wait until they check you in."

"Could you call Mary Lou tomorrow? She knows my kids' phone numbers."

"Of course."

I forgot to thank her then, but I will be grateful to Ann for the rest of my life. I think she knows that.

I don't remember when she left or when I was wheeled to my new hospital room. A dense fog seemed to settle on my brain. It was the beginning of many days of time warps and memory lapses.

Chapter 3

I Feel Like an Old Lady

"Why won't this stop," I whimpered, and then I retched. Darkness swirled around me as I tried to take a breath.

Where was I?

Like a tidal wave, the knowledge swept over me. The doctor said that I had metastasized cancerous tumors in my brain. They had decided to look for the source. The room spun, and I bent over a blue kidney-shaped dish and threw up again.

A cool, gentle hand rested on my back.

"Why won't this stop?" I asked again.

A young woman with short blonde hair used a washcloth to pat away the saliva around my mouth. Was she the ER nurse who had helped the doctor tell me I had cancer?

"The brain doesn't like to be messed with," she said.

I must have been given something to sleep. Time whirled away. I woke up once, and Ann appeared, a gentle visage, sitting on the window ledge like Grace Kelly at the end of the movie *Rear Window*, her long legs stretched out, a sweater over her shoulders, reading a magazine. I smiled to myself and fell back to sleep.

♦ ♦ ♦

"Dr. Ranch, call 316. Dr. Ranch, call 316."

My eyes opened slowly. Sunlight was flooding the large room. A rhythmic beeping of the heart monitor sounded in back of me.

Hmm, where was I?

A tall man with sandy-colored hair came in and smiled at me. "You're awake," he said as he picked up my wrist and looked at his watch.

Oh, right—the hospital.

I asked, "What time is it?"

"Around 8:00 a.m. I think. How are you feeling?"

"I'm actually hungry. What day is it anyway?"

"It's August 2. Do you know where you are?"

"Um. The hospital. Group Health. No that's not right." My face flushed. I couldn't remember the name.

"That's all right. It's Virginia Mason. Group Health contracts with us."

"Oh, okay. I can't believe I missed a whole day."

"You were pretty sick."

"It's just a big blank to me. What happened yesterday?"

"It looks like they did another CT, this time with contrast," he said, looking through the chart. "The results aren't back, but the doctor may have them when he comes around today."

He brushed my middle finger with an antiseptic swab and got out a small lancet.

"Just a little poke here." He squeezed out some blood and dripped it into a tube for a minute.

"That will do it." He put the blood sample away and peeled off his gloves. "Just call number five to order food. The Asian salad is pretty good."

As I held some cotton on my finger, I looked over the menu. This was the part of being in a hospital that I liked. No cooking, desserts any time I want, and even espresso drinks.

I looked up from the menu and stared into space. Why was I feeling so cheerful? I was acting like this was a big, beautiful hotel room and I was ordering breakfast in bed. They were looking for cancer in my body. I should be terrified.

I looked at the menu again, but I could make out nothing of what was written on it. Maybe the strong drugs that knocked me out yesterday were still in my system, making me kind of loopy and happy.

Perhaps I was in denial.

◆　◆　◆

There had been times in my past when I'd been very sick, and no one had known what to do. A feeling of fear and sense of desperation had first started to grow in me when I was twelve years old.

That summer of 1960 had been gorgeous. I lived in a small town east of Seattle, not far from Lake Washington. I loved going swimming every day, sleeping out under skies brilliant with layers of dazzling stars, and in the evening playing kick-the-can with the neighborhood kids.

One of my cherished pastimes was climbing the enormous pine tree across the street from my home. It was hundreds of years old, with resplendent emerald branches that were layered like the rungs of a ladder all the way to its top. While climbing I would breathe in the sharp fragrant smell of pine and my hands would become sticky with sap. Reaching the top, I could see houses and the Kirkland–Redmond highway far in the distance. Often the tree swayed gently in the wind, rocking me in its giant arms. I was never afraid of falling and liked leaning back against the trunk. It was absolutely still except for the breeze whispering through the pine needles and the lonesome sound of a distant car.

One day, climbing down the tree, I found that my leg wouldn't stretch out.

"Hey! What the heck's going on?"

I looked at my knees and both were slightly swollen, red, and hot to the touch.

I was alone and high up in a tree that hardly anyone walked under. What was I going to do? This was the first of many times I would ask that question.

Eventually by stretching out my leg and cautiously touching my toes and then placing my foot on the lower branch, I managed to find a way down. Safe at home, I said nothing, hoping the swelling would disappear on its own.

Yet the treacherous disease crept on, and my other joints began swelling. When I finally complained, my mom said, "You've got growing pains."

One night I woke up and felt that my body had turned to concrete. I could barely move my fingers and knees. It was pitch black in the cold, damp bedroom I shared with my little sister, who was asleep on the upper bunk.

"What's wrong with me?" I whispered to the darkness. I was too afraid to wake up Mom. Because then Dad might yell.

If I could just go to sleep, I'd be okay. I tried but kept waking up in pain.

♦ ♦ ♦

I kept complaining to my parents. Now that I've been a parent myself, I wonder why they didn't get me to a specialist right away. Perhaps there wasn't enough money for doctors.

Soon, I needed help getting dressed in the morning for school. Mom would turn on the hot water so I could hold my hands underneath the faucet and try to reduce the stiffness in my finger joints. After calling her to turn the faucet off, I'd hobble carrying my clothes into the living room and stand in the early morning darkness trying to get warm over the hot air vent. When I'd managed to get most of my clothes on, my mom would help pull up my nylons.

As my eighth grade continued, I started flunking PE. I couldn't run, jump hurdles, climb a rope to the ceiling, or even sit and get off the floor. I could barely bend my knees.

"Your knees are inflexible," my teacher pointed out one day.

I was flummoxed. I said nothing.

Toward the end of the first quarter, the teacher told me I could choose either a D or an F for my grade. Naturally, I chose a D—and accepted the subtle accusation that my lousy performance was my fault and that I was lucky not to flunk.

My mom and dad did not accept this poor mark on my report card. And when I told them the many reasons I'd received it, they finally called in a doctor.

He came to our home late one afternoon when the orange and gold maple leaves covered our yard. Opening his big black bag, he took out his thermometer and checked my temperature, looked at my tongue, and felt the heat of my swollen knees, fingers, and elbows. I told him how I was so stiff and walked so slowly at school that my classmates called me an "old lady."

I told him, "I yell back, 'I *feel* like an old lady.'"

The doctor smiled and eventually gave me a shot of antibiotics. I heard his quiet voice talking to my parents in the other room. He told them I probably had juvenile rheumatoid arthritis, and I'd most likely be in a wheelchair by age twenty. I was given vitamin C, aspirin, and antibiotics to take every day in case I had scarlet fever, which he thought could have caused the arthritis.

The pills I was taking gave me no relief, but gradually I learned to cope, hobbling up the dark rainy street to catch my school bus each morning, feeling a bit better as the day wore on, and always looking forward to getting home from school and hanging out with my friend, Barb.

♦   ♦   ♦

And I prayed. I prayed on Sundays sitting on the hard wooden pews of our Presbyterian church. I prayed at night before going to sleep, and one Christmas, stretched out face down on the floor, I prayed to the baby Jesus that lay under my little Christmas tree in my bedroom.

Finally, at age fifteen with my joints still inflamed, Dad sent me to another doctor who had an office in downtown Kirkland.

"Oh kid," the new doctor said, holding my swollen elbow, "we've got to do something for you. Oh kid, this isn't good."

He prescribed 5 milligrams of cortisone, and after a while the inflammation went away. I had no more pain and ceased waking in the dark nights worried about what was going to happen. I felt free. A smart doctor had come to my rescue, and I was safe. At least for a while.

I was eventually diagnosed with lupus, and there were many more times over the years that I was sick and sometimes ended up in the ER or hospital. I'd always recovered.

And now I was safe in a hospital surrounded by great technology and the best specialists.

They'd figure things out. If something went really wrong, they'd know what to do. I'd recovered before, and I would this time, too.

Chapter 4

WAITING FOR THE TESTS TO COME BACK

I had just finished breakfast when Mary Lou came in the room. "Mary Lou, you're here. I'm so relieved."

"Well, hello, dear," she said in her musical voice. She dropped her heavy purse on the floor. "Ann called me this morning. I am really so sorry to hear about your troubles."

"I know. I started talking in this kind of word salad at the meditation center and then ended up here," I said, gesturing around the room.

We talked on, cheerfully avoiding the subject of metastasized brain cancer.

"I called Alena. And she is calling Lily," Mary Lou said.

"Okay."

"They're going to try and reach you today and figure out when to come."

"When to come?"

"Yes, to help out."

"I don't know if they really need to."

She looked at me sharply and pulled up her chair. I had forgotten that Mary Lou had spent four years at Fred Hutchinson Cancer Research Center, helping on projects and sometimes dealing with cancer that had metastasized to the brain or liver. Like Ann, she knew what I was facing.

"It might be time to have them come, Susan."

I didn't know what to say. I remembered her words later, but at the time they didn't penetrate the dense fog in my brain.

"Oh, okay."

Sensing my reluctance, she said, "Well, we can talk about that later."

After a while Mary Lou left, promising to return in the evening.

My eyelids grew heavy, and I sank back on the pillow. For a long time, I heard Mary Lou talking outside of my room. I was glad to know that someone I knew and loved was close by.

The news of my illness tore around my family like a wildfire. Everyone was terrified and calling me, but my cell phone was dead and when my room phone rang, my blood was being drawn, my IV was being changed, or I was being rolled out of the room for another test.

The next day after a number of loud jangly rings, I was able to answer the room phone.

"Susan, this is your sis-in-law. I've been calling and calling you!"

"I'm sorry, Reva, it seems like I'm either getting tests or maybe out of the room when you call."

"Well, your brother and I want to come down to see you."

"Really? All this way?"

"Uh-huh, and afterward we'll drive up to the Ballard Locks and get some fish and chips."

"Earl's favorite Seattle place."

"That's right," she said, laughing.

We talked for a few minutes more about the locks, the hot weather, and hospital food. Reva promised a visit in a couple of days.

It was strange how our conversation was all about mundane, everyday things. Perhaps we were both clinging to a sense of safe normalcy, denying the existence of the edge of the dark abyss of a terminal disease that was appearing before us.

A few days passed with more tests. The worst of these was a spinal tap, in which they sucked the fluid out of my back. For a while afterward, I felt like I was a gas tank only three-quarters full. Luckily, this brought only a dull headache.

Every day, I waited for test results telling me where the cancer had originated. When they said all of the results were negative, I inwardly smiled. I still didn't believe I had cancer. I had always recovered, and I would this time too. I just knew it! Meanwhile, I visited with Mary Lou, talked with my kids on my newly recharged phone, and listened to the mantra.

◆　◆　◆

Toward the end of the week, Earl and Reva came to visit. My brother is eight years older and had always been a kind of hero to me. He was a rebel, of sorts, but when he was caught, our dad punished him with stinging blows from his belt. My brother refused to give Dad the satisfaction of crying out. My two sisters and I would hide in our bedroom, scared and feeling terrible for our brother.

That day in the hospital Earl and I walked arm in arm around the newly remodeled eighteenth floor. I realized that this was the oncology unit and that most of the other patients were seriously ill. Earl and I wanted to avoid seeing any of them, and so we walked down to the sunroom, with its tall palm plants, beige laminate floors, and enormous windows. To the west we could see a spectacular view of downtown Seattle all the way to Puget Sound, which was glittering in the sun. Tiny ferries were going in and out of the landing. To the north, far into the distance, construction workers were putting up new buildings for Amazon. Life went on.

Eventually, we sat down. I looked at my brother, with his bald head and a long black beard, dusted with gray. At one time, he'd had shiny, shoulder-length hair. He lost it all when he was treated with interferon for a year—a treatment for stage-three melanoma. The treatment had worked, but it caused all of the hair on his body to fall out. It had grown back everywhere but his head. I was just happy he was alive. He was a fighter.

Earl and I liked to talk about growing up in our family, and so now, feeling nostalgic, I asked him, "Do you remember when you ran away from home?"

He pushed his glasses up on his nose as if to see me better. "Dad always scared the crap out of me," he said. "Was that the time I was flunking junior high?"

"Yeah. I think Kenny came and told Mom."

It was a day in 1954. I remembered an urgent knock at our front door. Kenny, my brother's best friend, came to tell our mom that Earl had received a terrible report card and had run away. He had boarded a Greyhound bus and was going just as far as his fifteen dollars would take him.

My sister and I had huddled together on our faded green couch, listening to Mom telephoning our dad at work to tell him in her shaking voice about what Earl had done. I was only six, but I knew that this was a calamitous event. Dad said he'd drive to the Greyhound Bus Station and see if he could find out where Earl had gone.

Day had faded into night, and my mom prepared a dinner that no one ate. Finally, Dad came home. He said they'd figured out Earl had bought a ticket to Portland. The State Patrol had pulled over a bus heading in that direction—and Earl was on it. They were taking him to their office in Olympia. Mom was relieved and begged Dad not to be angry.

My sister and I chimed in, "Dad, please don't be mad at Earl. *Ple-e-e-ease!*"

Hearing this, back in the quiet sunroom at the hospital, Earl laughed, "Yeah, I was going to try and disappear on the streets of Portland. Dad wasn't exactly mad, but on the way home, he said, 'Next time, I'm going to let you just keep on going!'"

"You know what I did the next morning at school?" I asked. "I skipped down the sidewalk and sang, 'My brother ran awa-a-ay! My brother ran awa-a-ay.' I was proud of you and wished I had the courage that you had."

We got up and started walking back to the room.

"You have plenty of courage, Sis. You're going through all of this," he said, gesturing at the hospital hallway.

Then, like a car slowing to look at a horrendous accident, my eyes were drawn into a patient's room. I saw a wraith of a man, lying in a bed and connected to a dripping IV. His eyes were closed, his mouth open. My heart began to beat faster, and I sped up to get past this frightening image.

◆　◆　◆

When we got back to my room, a doctor was talking to Reva. They looked at me with solemn expressions.

Oh no! Had they found cancer?

The doctor spoke. "All of the test results are back." I held my breath. "We haven't found anything, so we recommend biopsy on one of the lesions in your brain."

Sitting down on the bed, I felt distanced from myself as if I was an actor on a stage doing a scene in a hospital room.

Finally, I managed to say, "It sounds like a logical step. Let's go ahead."

Little did I know what a fateful decision this would be.

Chapter 5

WHERE IS EVERYBODY?

"I'm there for you, Mom. I'll do anything you want. Just let me know."

My thirty-one-year-old daughter, Lily, was on the phone trying to reassure me, but her voice sounded high and taut, like a tightly pulled violin string.

"I really appreciate that, Sweetie. So far, my plan is to fly you out for the biopsy, and then you can be at home with me while we wait for the results. It looks like they're going to discharge me really soon from the hospital. I'll come back when the biopsy is scheduled. Afterward, I'll go back home again and wait for the results. So, that's when you could be with me. We can eat a lot and watch stupid TV shows. And it will be nice to have someone go to appointments with me."

"Whatever you want, Mom."

"Do you think you can get the time off?"

Lily had been working as wait staff in a restaurant in Missoula, Montana. They offered no paid time off. And she was living with a disabled veteran who couldn't work.

"I'll start looking for people to fill in for me so I can fly out right away. And since Alena is working and has Rowan to take care of, maybe she can come later."

"Yeah, but her bank gives her PTO. And since Ken has joint custody, maybe he can watch Rowan for a week or two." I took a long drink of water. I was getting tired. "Maybe you guys can figure it out."

Lily and I said our goodbyes, and I sank into my pillow. Even though I'd slept off and on the whole morning, I was exhausted. Just as I was drifting off, Mary Lou came in.

"Good morning, Susan," she said with a smile.

"Hi, Mary Lou. I just got off the phone with Lily. I'm going to make reservations for her to come and be with me during the biopsy and stay for a week or two."

"That's a great idea. I'm glad."

In that moment, my hospital internist appeared in the doorway with a look of urgency in his eyes.

"There's an opening in surgery early this afternoon," he said. "If you want, we can get you in for the biopsy."

"Really? Wow!"

Mary Lou and I looked at each other.

"Could you stay with me?" I asked Mary Lou.

"Of course. I don't want you to be alone, Susan."

"Thank you." I took her hand and gave it a squeeze. "Let's just get it over with."

Everything went into fast forward then, and before long I was being wheeled to the pre-op holding area.

Mary Lou and I sat in a small area partitioned off from the other people waiting for surgery. A nurse came in and stuck markers on my forehead and behind my ear.

"What are these?" I asked.

"They're called fiducials. They're markers to help align the MRI they took a few days ago to the image guidance system."

"I see." I had no idea what she was talking about.

"How are they getting the sample from her brain?" Mary Lou asked.

I held my breath, waiting for the answer.

"They will strip shave and prep the area on the left temporal part of her head, incise a small area of the scalp, and put a retractor into the incision. Then a high-speed drill will place a burr hole in her head. A navigation system will help guide the doctor so he can go in with the needle and get multiple specimens."

"When they're done, will my head just be stitched together?" I couldn't imagine how there would be enough skin on my scalp to do that.

"They have a cool little titanium miniplate they'll attach first with screws, and then they'll stitch you up." The nurse smiled as she left. "You'll be fine."

Once she was gone, I turned to Mary Lou. "I know they told me all of this when I signed the release forms. I must have blocked it out of my mind."

"It sounds pretty intense."

"I know! I can't get *burr hole* out of my head. Jeez!"

Time seemed to slow, and we became quiet listening to the hub-bub around us.

A lady in a bed across from me who had been talking to the nurse in a nervous high-pitched voice was finally wheeled away. In a short time, she was back, still talking but in a slow, groggy way.

Finally, a nurse came to get me.

"See you soon," I said, waving to Mary Lou.

I looked up at the yellow ceiling and blazing halogen lights as I was rolled down the hall to the operating room. When we arrived, I could see several people with surgical gowns and caps preparing the room.

Soon, a nurse put a clear mask over my nose and mouth. Startled I looked up at her.

"Breathe," she said.

I inhaled something biting that smelled like ozone and fell into an inky black abyss.

♦　♦　♦

Later I learned that the surgeon found Mary Lou in the pre-op cubicle and told her my surgery had gone really well. "We got several good samples," he said. "And Susan is in recovery right now."

Mary Lou found out what room I would be taken to—one on the seventh floor because everyone expected me to be going home the next day. She found the room then and, sitting down in it to wait for me, she thought, *Susan, you're not going to like this*! As a contrast to the spacious new room on the eighteenth floor, this space was cramped and well-worn, and I was sharing it with another patient, who had the window.

Once I was brought into the room, Mary Lou sat for a while longer, waiting for me to awaken.

Finally, a nurse came in to check my vitals and told her, "It may take some time for Susan to come out of the anesthetic. You might want to come back tomorrow."

Mary Lou set up photographs of our guru and of my daughters, and whispered into my ear, "We can visit in the morning."

As it turned out, it wasn't that easy.

◆　◆　◆

Someone was yelling in a scratchy demanding voice. I thrashed around in my bed, trying to throw off my tangled sheets and tell that person to shut up.

"You promised I would have a room by myself. Now I'm trapped in this crappy room with a roommate—AND WHERE THE HELL IS THE WINDOW!"

A warm, soft hand came to rest on my forearm. I looked at it and peered up to see the face that came with the hand. Was she the one who was yelling?

"After your biopsy, they put you here for some reason," a melodious voice said. "Let's see if I can get a nurse to move you." The person speaking was an attractive older woman with dark hair streaked with grey. Her eyes, light blue, looked at me with concern. Then she left the room.

As she stepped away, this woman opened a curtain for a moment. On the other side, a scowling woman was lying in another bed.

What was *her* problem?

I hollered, "GET ME OUT OF HERE!"

It seemed that I was the one doing the yelling.

◆　◆　◆

The room was warm and stuffy. It had pale-yellow walls, and the sun was streaming in the window, making pools of light on the floor.

It was so warm.

I tried to push off the blanket. I felt flooded with nausea. I shut my eyes tightly to make it go away.

◆　◆　◆

"Good morning," said a man in a white jacket.

"Good morning," I said, letting a smile crinkle my face.

He got very close and shone a flashlight into my eyes. He had rimless glasses and warm brown eyes. His hair was jet black and greying at the temples. Was he saying something to me? His lips were moving, and sound was coming from his mouth. He was so nice, and I tried saying something back, but I was so tired.

"Ouch, ouch, OUCH!" He was sticking something into my foot. I moved my feet up under the bedcovers to get them away from him.

He pointed at his nose, so I pointed at mine. He was *so* nice. I wanted to be a good student. He squeezed my hands, and I squeezed back. He smiled so I must have done a good job.

I blinked, and he was gone.

I guess I fell asleep.

I opened my eyes, and Mary Lou was sitting in the chair.

"Do you like your new room, Susan?"

I blinked, and she disappeared too. I looked around. It was night outside, and I was all alone. A chill ran down my body.

Where *was* everybody?

A young woman appeared out of nowhere and was talking to me in a sing-song voice like I was a child. She was pushing on my back.

"Ow, ow, OW!!!" I thrashed and batted my hands at her.

Why wouldn't she leave me alone. I wasn't a child! She should just go away.

I lay on my side and drew my knees to my chest. I squeezed my eyes shut and the first line of an old childhood verse ran through my mind over and over again.

I'm hiding, I'm hiding. I'm somewhere inside…

This is the last conscious thought I had for quite a while. I wrote the next five chapters from conversations I had later with my daughters, my sister, and my friends who *were* conscious of what was happening to me while I was not. I was also able to ask a few of my doctors to help me make sense of my medical records during this time. For a couple of weeks, there was no "I" to observe and tell my story.

Chapter 6

ALENA: WHY IS MOM ACTING THIS WAY?

Alena was terrified. Her mother was lying in a fetal position, gurgling, moaning, saying, "Pain, pain, pain," staring off into space... When the doctor tapped her mom's knee to check her reflexes, she turned away from him and yelled, "Ow, ow, OW!"

"It's okay, Mom," Alena said in what she hoped was a compassionate voice. "Try and do what the doctor wants you to. He's here to help you."

To the doctor, she said, "I'm sorry. I don't understand what's going on with her—why she's acting like this. Is it the pain?"

The doctor—Alena thought he was an internist—looked down at her mother's medical chart. "Some people experience a sort of delirium after surgery," he said, "or even just from being in the hospital—although she hasn't been here that long." He paused. "We can give her something for the pain. But we'll need to discontinue some of her other meds—like Ambien—which might be contributing to the delirium."

He added, "It's good that her brain biopsy came back as negative."

Alena was shocked. "What! You mean she doesn't have cancer? We were told she likely had metastatic cancer in her brain! Does this mean there's no cancer in her body?"

He hesitated for a minute. "Not exactly." His pager went off, and he closed the chart and stood up to leave. "She's had another lumbar puncture, and as soon as we get the results back, we will know more. Dr. Fink should be in soon, and he can explain more." Seeing her confusion, he said, "The oncologist."

After the internist left, her mom fell asleep. Alena was exhausted herself, and she could feel a headache coming on. She tried massaging the tight knots in her forehead. Finding some ibuprofen in her purse, she dry-swallowed three of them.

She grabbed a comb, walked to the mirror, and tried untangling her long curly brown hair.

"What a mess," she said to herself.

Mary Lou had dropped her off at the hospital early, and there had been no time to straighten it or put on makeup. She looked for mascara.

◆ ◆ ◆

Mary Lou came in and set down her capacious flowered purse.

"Hi Mary Lou," Alena said. "You're back."

"Hi Alena. How's your mom doing today?"

"She's been in a lot of pain."

Alena told her about the biopsy results.

"Oh my gosh, that's great news."

A doctor with a grey beard and wispy hair came briskly in the room.

"I'm Dr. Fink," he said, shaking Alena's hand with a pleasant smile.

She looked at him blankly for a moment. "Oh, right," she said, "you're the oncologist. I'm Susan's youngest daughter, Alena."

"I think we've met," said Mary Lou.

"Yes," he said. "You're the sister."

Alena hid a smile. Early on, Mary Lou had said she was her mom's sister to get needed medical information.

"Let's find another room so we can talk," he said.

Alena's stomach dropped. She and Mary Lou looked at each other. What now?

Dr. Fink led them to an empty room with three comfortable chairs pulled in a circle. They sat down quietly.

"Susan has lymphoma."

Alena's heart sped up and her mouth went dry. Mary Lou took hold of Alena's hand and asked the doctor some questions. Alena looked at the floor, not hearing a word of what was said. Her mother had *lymphoma!* They'd just said she didn't have brain cancer, and now they were saying she had lymphoma.

Alena tried to focus on what the doctor was telling Mary Lou. ". . .We need the final test results from the spinal tap to absolutely confirm, but I wanted you to be prepared."

After the doctor left, the two women sat silently for a few minutes.

Mary Lou spoke first. "I'm just stunned," she said.

"Me too." Alena ran a hand over her forehead. "God, I am just so exhausted right now."

May Lou looked at her sadly. "Why don't you go down to the coffee shop, and I'll go back to the room and be with your mom." Then she added one bright afterthought: "The test results aren't in yet, so there's still a chance she's okay."

♦   ♦   ♦

Alena took an elevator to the cafeteria for a much-needed break. Standing in line to pay for her drink, she picked up a flyer advertising Al-Anon meetings.

I could have used this a long time ago, she thought with a wry smile. She sat down with her cup of coffee, and thoughts of her soon-to-be ex-husband crept, unwanted, into her mind. Ken had received a citation for driving drunk the first year they were married. She'd bailed him out of jail, hired a lawyer, and had gone to court with him for what turned out to be the first of many times.

At his most recent court hearing, the judge had given Ken a hefty fine, an ankle bracelet that confined him to their apartment, and an alcohol ignition interlock device to use when he drove to work. Ken had to breathe into the interlock device, and if there was no alcohol on his breath, he was able to start the car. The equipment wasn't provided by the court, and it wasn't cheap, either. It had cost them a lot. Ken had also been ordered to go to ten AA meetings. He hated these meetings. He said that all the talk about a "higher power" made him feel desolate inside.

The entire ordeal had cost thousands of dollars and stressed their fledgling marriage to the breaking point. Alena had sworn to Ken that if he ever got another DUI, she'd leave him.

◆ ◆ ◆

To save money, they'd rented the studio apartment in the downstairs of her mom's house.

Things had started to get better, but then she'd gotten pregnant. After Rowan was born, Ken had started drinking heavily again. He'd been working on a government contract, and when that ended, which it did, he was unemployed. Depressed and angry, Ken started staying up all night, drinking whiskey, and playing video games. He'd taken some online courses using the GI Bill, but he didn't complete any of them. At Alena's insistence, he applied for jobs all over the country and finally received an offer in Lincoln, Nebraska.

Alena vividly remembered her mother's shock when she told her the news.

"You're moving where?" her mom had asked, her voice sounding brittle.

"Nebraska. Lincoln, Nebraska."

"Nebraska? Why?"

"Ken got a job, Mom. Isn't that great? And the houses are so cheap there we can actually afford to buy one. I'll be able to stay home with Rowan, and he can start kindergarten in the fall. Isn't that great?"

"Yeah. I guess it's good news. When are you moving?"

"Right after Thanksgiving."

"But that's only three weeks!"

"I know. I just couldn't tell you, Mom."

"Well, at least we can have one final Thanksgiving together."

"We're having Thanksgiving dinner at Dad's," Alena said quietly. Her parents had divorced years before, and they had never developed a friendly rapport.

"So, no Thanksgiving, no Christmas," her mom's voice cracked.

"Well, you can come visit."

Alena had felt terrible, but at the time, it seemed like she had no choice.

◆　◆　◆

Soon, Alena left family and friends behind to try to save her floundering marriage and fulfill her dreams of being a stay-at-home mom. She had spent her first Christmas in Lincoln with below-zero temperatures and the unceasing Nebraska wind rattling the shutters of their new house.

One night, in late January, her hopes for a fresh start came crashing to an end with a telephone call from her husband. He was in jail. He'd been arrested for driving while drunk. It was his third DUI. Alena was ashamed. She told no one but her sister. Had she made a terrible mistake moving to Nebraska? Alena closed herself off from her husband, refusing to accept his apologies or offer warmth or support of any kind. His own mother had hired an attorney for him and paid his court costs. The judge ordered him to stop drinking and to go into counseling.

Once again, the remedy didn't work. Ken had started drinking and taking drugs in high school. He'd never learned to solve problems or deal with negative emotions. He didn't like going to group counseling, and he blamed any difficulties in their marriage on Alena. She expected too much of him.

Susan had come to visit in March, for her grandson's birthday. Alena knew her mom suspected something was terribly wrong. Susan commented that Ken wouldn't even make eye contact with her and that her grandson kept pretending he was Peter Parker and, over and over again, he kept finding ways to rescue his mom. Alena had made excuses, saying Rowan missed his Memaw—his grandmother—and all of his friends from his preschool back home in Washington.

In late April, thinking a break would be good for everyone, Alena took Rowan to Florida to visit his other grandmother. Alena felt the sun and beach would be healing for both of them. Her mother-in-law worked every day, but Alena relaxed by her pool and took videos of a confident Rowan learning to swim.

On Mother's Day, in May, Alena phoned her mom from Florida. "Happy Mother's Day," she said, her voice set in an artificial cheerfulness.

"Hi, Sweetie! Happy Mother's Day to you too. Are you enjoying your day?"

Alena started to tell her mom about how Rowan had learned to swim, when she saw there was a call waiting from her husband. He had been calling every other day, yelling at her that any problems they had were her fault.

"Can I call you back in a few minutes?"

"Okay, talk to you in a while."

♦ ♦ ♦

Alena picked up the call from Ken and got right to the point, "Why are you calling again?"

Ken asked, "Have you called the new counselor?"

"What counselor?"

"The group counseling isn't working for me, Alena. I have to go to a new one, or I'll go back to jail and go fucking nuts. Why don't you get this?"

"Why don't you call the counselor yourself?" she yelled.

"You know I can't call and make appointments. I have social anxiety. It's easy for you. And why are you with my mother? Bring Rowan back. He's my only source of love."

"How do you think that makes me feel? Like a piece of crap! So, call the new counselor yourself."

Alena hung up then and called her mom back. She almost told her mother about Ken's new DUI, but she was still feeling too ashamed to say anything. Still, she had to explain something of what was going on with her husband.

"Mom," she said, "Ken has stopped drinking, which is good, but he's blaming me for all the emotions he can't bury anymore. And he wants me to fix everything."

"I'm so sorry, Sweetie. I'm glad that he's finally stopped drinking, but he has to make a steady effort every single day so he can get better. We all have to work on ourselves. It's not up to you to straighten out Ken." She added, "Honey, you deserve so much more."

Alena started sobbing then. She finally said, "I just want to be happy."

Sounding terrified, her mother said, "I feel like I'm going to lose you, like you're teetering on the edge of an abyss! The only thing I can think of is for you to find an Al-Anon group. It really helped me understand my family and your dad."

"I know," Alena choked back her tears. "I'll be all right. Maybe tomorrow will be a better day." She knew Al-Anon was a good idea, but she never seemed to have the time for it.

◆　◆　◆

In September, Alena went to New York to help with her best friend's wedding. She was inspired by the many people her age who had successful careers. Alena especially liked the groom's best friend. He was a buyer for his parents' bookstore in New York City and a recovering alcoholic. She told him all about Ken. They talked for many hours, and he was respectful and compassionate.

Back home in Nebraska, Alena was ready to keep trying with her marriage but unwilling to cut off all communications with her new friend. They emailed each other and texted almost every day. One day her husband confronted her.

"Alena, who the hell is this?" he yelled. He was holding Alena's phone in the air, open to the texts from her friend.

"It's just a friend of Suzanna's. He's a buyer for a bookstore, and we text about books. Give me my phone back. Right now, Ken."

"You slept with him, didn't you?" he said, his face only an inch from hers.

"Nothing happened! We just talk about books."

Her head pounding with a migraine, she finally grabbed Rowan, ran to her bedroom, and locked the door. Ken banged on the door, scaring his five-year-old son.

The confrontations went on daily. Alena had chronic headaches and couldn't stop shaking. Finally, in early October, she told Ken she couldn't take it anymore and was done with their marriage. He had started taking medication for anxiety and panic attacks, but it did not calm his explosive and erratic behavior.

One afternoon after he'd been following her around screaming, Alena threw some random clothes into a bag, wrestled her phone back from Ken, caught hold of Rowan, and ran for the car. She drove for a while and then pulled over and called her mom. As she told her what had happened, Rowan sat silently staring out the window.

"Ken keeps texting me, Mom. He says he's going to call the police if I don't bring Rowan back right now."

"Do not go back there, Alena," her mother told her. "You and Rowan both could be in danger. Do you have the number for the free women's attorney we found you? Go there right now."

The attorney had told her she was doing nothing illegal and to tell her husband that she was taking some time away. The attorney also advised Alena to take the batteries out of her phone because otherwise her husband could track her and also track all of her phone calls. Alena needed to get a new phone and a place to stay. Unfortunately, the shelter had an eight-week waiting list. Alena was unemployed and had no friends in the area.

But her mom was fiercely protective. First, she'd called around Lincoln and found a place where Alena and Rowan could stay. A few days later, Susan flew to Lincoln and stayed for seven weeks. Alena smiled to herself as she remembered her mom coming down the escalator at the Lincoln Airport terminal. She'd never been so happy to see her mother's face. Susan had helped her find a good attorney, a new job, and an apartment. Rowan loved visiting his Meemaw, playing, and going to movies.

♦ ♦ ♦

Alena finished her coffee and began walking back to the hospital room. After a great deal of marriage counseling, Alena felt she had tried her best but, sadly, the marriage was not going to work. Now, she was a nearly divorced single mom, had new friends, and even went on an occasional date.

She took an elevator to the busy seventh floor.

"Your turn, Mary Lou," she said as she entered the room.

"Okay, I won't be long. Susan seems to be getting a little restless. So, I'll grab some food and be right back."

Alena sat down by the bed. Her mother started groaning.

"Mum, are you okay?"

Her mom's eyes flew open.

"Pain, pain," she cried, pointing to her head.

Alena stroked her cheek and said, "I'm here. I'm here. I'll never let you go. Remember I used to say that to you when I was little? I mean it. I'll never let you go."

She buzzed for the nurse again. Why the hell haven't they brought her any pain medicine?

"Pa-a-a-a-a-ain! A string on the mound. Please. Please," she bawled. "Buy the groceries favaforgo."

This wasn't making sense! "I need help in here," Alena shouted. No one came.

Frantically she looked around the room for something to help. Her eyes fell on the guru's picture.

Alena picked up the photo and looked at it. A quietness settled over her like a winter's snowfall. She felt compelled to assure her mom that the guru was there protecting her. Tears welled up in her eyes.

"Mum, the guru is with you. She loves you. I love you too." She repeated this like a mantra.

Gradually her mom breathed easier. Tears streamed down Alena's cheeks. Somehow, everything would be all right.

A nurse came into the room and turned off the call button. "Yes, can I help you?"

Alena gathered her strength and said, "My mom just had a brain biopsy, and she needs more pain meds. Right now."

"The doctor is right next door, doing rounds. I'll go get him."

"Thank you so much."

Alena held her mom's hand. "You've always been there for me. You have fought for me over and over. Now, it's my turn."

Chapter 7

ALENA & LILY: WILL SHE EVER COME HOME?

A hand smacked Lily in the face.

"Ouch! What the hell?" she mumbled, rubbing her nose.

It was early morning, and golden sunlight streamed through the window. She had arrived in Seattle late the night before, and she was tired and disoriented.

Who had hit her? "Matt?" she said quietly, feeling the body next to her.

"Hey, get your hand off my butt!"

"Oops, sorry," Lily said. "I thought you were Matt."

Alena giggled. "You're lucky it's me. The both of you would never fit in this bed."

They were in their mom's guest room, having decided the night before that sleeping in her empty queen-size bed was too creepy.

Lily yawned and turned over on her back.

"I didn't know where I was when I woke up. I thought I was home with Matt sleeping next to me. That's a laugh. He can't sleep, so he plays video games all night. You smacked me in the face, by the way."

"Sorry, I was really restless. God, I'm exhausted. Not sure I'm ready for a long flight back."

Lily fluffed up her pillow and sat up in bed. A sweet summer breeze ruffled the curtains.

Alena turned over on her side and looked at her sister.

"We haven't seen each other for two years, and now you're going home," Lily said.

"I know, and under this circumstance too."

"We haven't talked about Mom much."

Alena looked off into the distance, her eyes seeing nothing. "I need to wake up first," she said.

"Why don't I make some coffee."

"Okay. I want to call Rowan to tell him I'll be seeing him tonight."

Lily wandered into the kitchen. She found the coffee pot and a bag of coffee, which was in the freezer. As the coffee perked, she walked into the living room. The house felt forlorn and empty. Running her hand along the striped rose and tan love seat, she walked up to the fireplace. There were three framed batiks sitting on the mantle. Her favorite was of a woman who seemed to be dancing in the clouds. She picked up a small, surprisingly heavy pale green elephant sitting next to it. Her mom loved African art and had been on a safari to Botswana, Zambia, and Zimbabwe. Lily sighed and put the elephant back.

Her mom loved all this stuff. Would she ever come home?

A little later, Lily and Alena sat out on the deck, enjoying the morning sun. Somewhere in the backyard a nuthatch called, sounding like a nasal tin horn. Chickadee babies bravely ate at a suet bird feeder that hung from the eaves in front of the kitchen window.

"Who's going to feed the birds?" Lily asked.

"Who's going to feed the cat?" Alena added. "Diane loves him so maybe you can walk across the street, knock on her door, and ask her to. I don't know her phone number."

"Okay, so prepare me for seeing Mom. Has she woken up at all?" Lily asked.

"Not really. She just lies in bed curled up in a fetal position. Sometimes she garbles out some words, but usually nothing anybody can understand—except for 'pain.' She says that a lot. She was in so much pain yesterday, it was awful."

Alena stared at Lily and chewed on the corner of her lip.

"Jesus, why won't she wake up?" Lily asked, her voice becoming shrill. "What do the doctors say?"

"The biopsy results came back negative."

"What?"

"Yeah. Guess it's good she doesn't have a cancerous malignancy in her brain," Alena said ruefully. "So now they're doing more tests." She didn't have the courage to mention the real possibility of lymphoma.

Lily rubbed her eyes. "Poor Mom."

Alena blew on her hot coffee to cool it. "One day I read her one of the guru's smaller books. When I finished, she opened her eyes and said, 'I love you.'"

Lily closed her eyes and swallowed the tears that were rising in her throat. "I wish you could stay longer."

"What am I going to do, Lily? I have to go back to work, and I can't leave Rowan too long with Ken."

"I know. I'll get all the information I can from the doctors and try to find out what's going *on* with her. And let's stay in touch somehow."

"It's hard when I'm at work ten hours a day." Alena sighed and put her coffee down on the table. "We've got to get ready. Mary Lou will drop you off at the hospital and take me right to the airport."

They scooted their chairs back from the picnic table.

"What if I never see her again?" Alena asked in a sorrowful voice. "We're too young to lose our mother."

Chapter 8

LILY: WHY WON'T SHE WAKE UP?

Lily could not understand what had happened to her mother. Just a few days ago, they'd talked on the phone. Her mom had made Lily's plane reservations so she could come and help after the biopsy. And now her mom was curled up on the hospital bed in a fetal position with her eyes shut tightly. Every once in a while, she'd moan and thrash about. And that was it! That was all she did! What was happening!

Lily looked at where the IV tubes had left dark blue bruises on her mother's thin wrist. She said, "Your poor wrists."

Her mom opened her eyes and said, in a scratchy tremulous voice, "Love."

"I love you too, Mum! Are you awake?" Lily buzzed for a nurse. "Are you thirsty? Can I get you something?"

Her mother pointed to her head. "Hurt," she said.

"Hurt? Your head hurts? I know it's because of the biopsy. The nurse is coming. We'll get you something."

Her mother closed her eyes, groaned, and flailed her arms.

"I love you, Mom."

Feeling helpless and close to tears Lily stood up and walked to the window. It was another clear sunny day, and she could see all the way to downtown Seattle. Her mom had finally gotten a private room with a big window. There were flowers and cards from friends sitting on the sill.

Lily pushed back her long auburn hair and opened a card with a striped umbrella and a "Get Well" message written across it: "The best way to stop these silly cards from coming is to *get well*."

Lily smiled, knowing there had been many cards from this particular friend. Maybe one a day her mother *would* get well.

"Can I help you?"

Lily turned around to see a petite brunette in blue scrubs standing at the door. "I'm Sharon, Susan's nurse for today."

"Oh hi. I'm Lily, her oldest daughter. I flew in from Montana last night. My sister had to go home. I called you just now because my mom seemed to wake up for a moment. She said, 'love' and 'hurt.'" Lily's voice shook with emotion. "Then she closed her eyes and went back to thrashing her arms and legs all over. I want to know what's wrong with her. Why won't she wake up?"

Sharon looked at Lily sympathetically. "Just a moment, and I'll go get her chart."

Lily walked to the door and watched Sharon go to the nurse's station. They were on the seventh floor, in the neurology ward. The walls were an unappealing mustard color, and the fluorescent lights bothered her eyes. But it was very quiet for a hospital, and that at least was good.

Sharon returned, looking through the notes on her mom.

"The results from the spinal tap came back and, the good news is, she doesn't have lymphoma."

Lily caught her breath, "What?" she managed to squeeze out. "They thought she had lymphoma!"

"Yes, that was the working diagnosis. But she does not."

"Well, that's good, I guess."

"She's also had another MRI." Sharon flipped through some pages. "I don't see the results yet, but the doctor should have them by now." She looked at the white board on the wall, which listed Lily's mother's statistics, nurse, and doctor.

"It's Dr. H. I saw him earlier, so he should come shortly."

"Why is my mom so agitated?"

"Most likely it's because she has edema, a swelling, in her brain. That often causes a sort of delirium. And the symptoms are exactly what we're seeing in your mother—agitation, combativeness, confusion. It looks like they attempted another MRI, but the first time she was distressed. She wouldn't, or couldn't, be still enough for them to get any results. The next time they were successful, so you should know more soon."

Lily asked more questions and learned that her mother was being given both antiviral and antifungal medications to see if either of them helped. The nurse had used the word "empirically"; she said that the medications had been initiated "empirically." So, that meant they were doing it to see what worked. In other words, they didn't know. It was certainly weird to think that there might be a fungus growing in Mom's brain.

Sharon closed up the chart and looked around the room. She said, "It's peaceful in here. I like that music."

Lily hesitated for a second. "Oh, you mean the mantra. It's our guru singing the mantra."

"It's nice," Sharon said.

A short time later a man came in and introduced himself as Dr. H. He had black curly hair, blue eyes, and olive skin. Lily wondered if he was Armenian.

The doctor went over some test results with her. Lily was alarmed when she found out her mother's white blood cell count (CD4 on the chart), was 65, when the normal range would be between 500 and 1,500. Thank God, her test for HIV had been negative.

"We discontinued her mycophenolate. It's a drug your mother was taking for lupus that was most likely suppressing her white blood count. People with organ transplants have to take it so their body doesn't reject their new organ. We're taking her off it, so her CD4 should come up."

"Will she be okay without it?"

"For now."

Then he went over the latest MRI results. It was bad. The lesions in her mother's brain were spreading. Worse yet, there was increasing hemorrhage in the left temporal and frontal areas of her brain.

"Oh my God," Lily said. "You mean her brain is still bleeding? That's terrible. It's not cancer, so what's causing this?"

"Right now, we don't know."

Lily hugged herself tightly. Her breath caught in her throat.

"But we're keeping a close eye on her, and the infectious disease specialist and neurologist are consulting. They'll stop by and talk to you soon. They may have more test results."

After the doctor left, Lily sat and looked at her mom with tears in her eyes. She started thinking, "Don't die, Mom. Don't die!"

Chapter 9

LILY & JOANNE: THEY ALMOST LOST HER LAST NIGHT!

L ily drove slowly through the winding roads of the arboretum on her way to Mary Lou's house in Madison Valley. Early morning bike riders rode toward her on their way to work or getting in some exercise before another blazingly hot day. She remembered many trips with Alena and their mom to see Mary Lou and her daughter, Suzanna. Sometimes they'd all go down the hill to Madison Park to swim in Lake Washington; sometimes the kids would play dress-up and act out stories for their moms.

A wave of sadness swept over Lily. There might never be a time when they all would be together again. Or if they were, would it be at her mother's funeral?

"Stop thinking that," Lily said aloud. She struggled to focus on something else.

Aunt Boo Boo and Uncle Louie were coming today—for the first time since Mom got sick!

A shiver went through Lily when she thought of how her mom had looked yesterday: connected to tubes, curled up in bed, and mumbling incoherently.

What were Aunt Boo Boo and her husband going to think?

Still, it would be great to see them. Aunt Boo Boo—her mother's older sister, JoAnne—had always been a part of Lily's life. Their families visited each other every three or four months. One of Lily's favorite childhood memories was when her artistic aunt would pull out paint and brushes and little wooden boxes, bird houses, or various trinkets for the kids to decorate. Often, Lily and her sister and mother would make a quick trip to the Oregon Coast to see Aunt Boo Boo and family and to walk along the beach collecting shells, eating giant ice cream cones, and playing in the arcade.

Lily turned down Mary Lou's tree-lined street and then pulled to a stop in front of her blue grey house. Looking in the visor mirror, she was surprised to find that tears had smeared her mascara. She spit on her index finger and vigorously rubbed the skin underneath her eyes until the black smudges lessened. She didn't want Mary Lou to know she'd been crying.

They took Mary Lou's car to the hospital. As she drove, Mary Lou asked in her calm, reassuring voice whether JoAnne would be coming to the hospital today.

"Yeah," Lily said, "I'm excited to see her. Aunt Boo Boo had a long talk with Dr. H, and now she feels a lot better about Mom."

"Let's hope it stays that way."

"Right," Lily said taking a deep breath. "Let's hope."

◆　◆　◆

Someone was weeping.

Lily rounded the corner into her mother's room.

"Aunt Boo Boo? You're here. What's wrong?"

Her mother's older sister was crumpled in a chair next to the bed.

"The nurse said they almost lost her last night," she choked out, tears streaming down her face.

Lily's head swam with confusion. She sat down and put her arm around her aunt. "What? Lost who? Mom? No one told me that." Lily looked out the door for a moment. "Mary Lou stopped at the nurse's station. Maybe they'll tell her something."

"And look at her," JoAnne cried, turning from her niece to look at again at her sister. "She looks just awful."

Susan was lying on her side in a fetal position, her head tucked in, and her knees pulled up to her chest. Lily gently drew the blanket up around her mother's shoulders. Still, she looked vulnerable and exposed.

"I just don't understand," JoAnne said. "Yesterday, I had a nice long phone call with Susie's doctor. He made me feel so much better. He said they were doing all these tests, and they were definitely going to figure out what was wrong with her. Then I talked to Father Edmond, and he told me that God is with me and that Susie will be all right. I had been telling him that God had deserted me, but Father just laughed and said that the Lord is always with me. When Louie and I left home this morning, I was so excited about seeing my sister again."

JoAnne paused a moment, and Lily squeezed her hand.

"You just can't imagine how shocked I was when we got here, and the nurse said that they'd just about lost her last night. And then, when I saw her, looking like this—not even able to recognize me. Not even able to talk! I was shocked—and Louie couldn't take it." She said looked over her shoulder. "He just left. I'm not sure where he is."

"I don't know what the hell that nurse meant," Lily said. Then she remembered that her aunt did not like swearing. "Oops!" she added. "Sorry Aunt Boo Boo."

"That's okay," JoAnne said, taking a shaky breath. Swearing was the least of their problems. The two of them sat for a few minutes listening to the quiet voices in the hall and occasional paging of doctors.

When Mary Lou came in, she had obviously not heard anything more from the nurses. After saying hello to JoAnne, Mary Lou asked how Susan was doing today.

Lily answered: "She's been sleeping pretty quietly—since I've been here, anyway." Lily looked at JoAnne.

"She was agitated when I first saw her," JoAnne said, "She didn't even know who I was. I was horrified. And, as I told Lily, Louis left. That was a couple of hours ago. She's been like this for most of that time. One of the nurses told me they almost lost her last night. She almost died! Did the nurses say anything about that to you?"

Mary Lou shook her head. "They said they're waiting for more test results."

"I did some research last night on the internet," Lily said. "With her suppressed immune system and the fact that she has a cat I thought she might have toxoplasmosis. I got so excited that I called the doctor. He called me back and said they'd already tested for that, and the results were negative. As well as listeria and histo...something."

"Histoplasmosis," Mary Lou said.

"What's that," JoAnne asked.

"It's a type of lung infection inhaled from fungal spores from bird or bat droppings. I had told the doctor Susan had gone to Africa a couple of years ago, but those results were negative also," Mary Lou continued.

Lily pressed her hands onto her eyes and breathed in and out slowly. "Let's put on the mantra."

The guru's resonant, sweet voice permeated the air, and everyone grew quiet. All eyes were on Susan. Was she going to wake up? And if she did, would she even be Susan anymore?

◆ ◆ ◆

The morning wore on, with the nurses changing IV's and checking vitals. Friends from Susan's work and the meditation center came in and sat for a while, some quietly praying or saying the mantra.

Finally, Dr. H arrived with an assistant, introducing himself to JoAnne.

"Oh, I remember you," JoAnne said in a chirpy, bird-like voice. "We had a long phone conversation. You were so positive."

"JoAnne's kind of worried about the way my mom looks now," Lily explained to the doctor. "She doesn't seem to recognize people, she's agitated, and. . ." Feeling like her throat was closing, Lily let her words trail off.

JoAnne finished for her. "Like she's in a coma or something!"

"I feel like we're in a kind of limbo, waiting for these elusive test results," Lily managed to say.

"I understand how it seems like that," the doctor said. "We're consulting with the UW hospital. And I know Dr. Thottingal, the infectious disease specialist, is talking to them also. Susan has been on acyclovir, an antiviral, for almost three weeks now, so we might begin to see results from that." Sitting on the bed, right next to Susan, he turned to his assistant and said, "Let's try to sit her up."

The assistant raised the bed, and she and the doctor propped Susan up.

Susan did not seem to like this. "Hu-r-r-rt," she whined. "Ow-w-w-w."

"Hi," Dr. H said to her. "Do you know where you are?" When she gave no response, he asked, "Who's this?" he said with his hand on Lily's arm.

"Love," Susan said, a smile flitting across her face."

"Love you, Mom," Lily said, taking hold of Susan's pale hand.

"Hi Susie," JoAnne said. "I'm so happy to see you."

Susan did not look at her sister, but the doctor didn't follow up on that. "Can you follow this light?" he asked Susan, moving the beam from a tiny flashlight slowly, side to side, across her eyes.

This got a response. Susan started yelling, "UHHHHHH! OW OW! HURT!" She slumped down then and began thrashing her head back and forth.

"Oh no," JoAnne whispered.

"Mom, settle down, settle down," Lily said, stroking her arm.

"Well, it looks like she's not up to following directions," Dr. H said cheerfully, clicking off his flashlight. "Maybe we'll try this later."

Looking at the chart on his clipboard, he told them an MRI was scheduled soon, and that this would, hopefully, give them more information.

"Like what?" Lily asked.

"Well, the acyclovir should be having an effect by now. The test will let us know whether or not it's working."

But what if it isn't working? Lily bit her lip to avoid putting into words the dismal thought that crossed her mind. She hoped that her aunt wasn't feeling the same sense of dread she was.

Dr. H ordered more pain medication, and soon it was administered by a nurse. Before long, Susan was sleeping.

Feeling claustrophobic, Lily said that she was going to get some fresh air.

Her aunt asked, "Can I join you?"

"Of course," Lily said, and then she invited Mary Lou to join them.

"I need to get going now," Mary Lou said. "I'll be back early this evening."

Chapter 10

Lily & JoAnne: Bye Bye Blackbird

As the three of them took the elevator down to the lobby, Lily realized she was having trouble breathing. She wondered if she were having an anxiety attack. She thought, *That's all I need right now.* Then Lily realized that maybe she was upset because of the story from that phantom nurse who'd said that they had "almost lost" her mom. As soon as the elevator door opened, Lily walked rapidly outside to the hospital's courtyard. The fresh air helped. She had to not let herself be upset by rumors!

JoAnne said, "Sweetie, could you get me a cookie while I try to track Louie down on my cell phone?"

Refreshments sounded like an excellent plan. Lily gathered some sweets, and then she sat outside in the shade, waiting for her aunt. Just sitting outside began to revive her.

Eventually, JoAnne showed up with the news that her husband was sitting in their car. Picking up her outsize chocolate chip cookie with relish, JoAnne said, "Louie can't face seeing your mom this way."

"I can understand," Lily said, taking a sip of her coffee.

"If your grandmother were here, she would sing."

"Sing?"

"Whenever we were upset, she said, 'Let's sing.' And we would start crooning the songs she grew up with. Things like 'I'm Looking Over a Four Leaf Clover' and 'Bye Bye Blackbird.'"

Lily *did* know them. "Mom would sing those songs too, with us kids. She loves the song she did in the neighborhood talent show when she was a kid—you know, the one that starts, 'Pack up all my cares and woe, here I go, swingin' low. . .' I don't know if that's it for sure, but it's close."

"What about if we get your mom singing? Maybe that would trigger her brain or something."

"That's an idea," Lily said. "In fact, it's a *great* idea. I've read that singing helps patients with aphasia. And that's what Mom seems to have, for sure."

◆　◆　◆

Late that afternoon the physical therapist got Susan sitting up in bed.

"I'm going to leave for a while and see if she can stay sitting up," the nurse told JoAnne and Lily. "I'll be back in about twenty minutes."

Once the nurse was gone, Lily said, "Why don't we try singing now." She turned to Susan and said, "Mom, hi. Can you open your eyes?"

Susan peered at her daughter through little slits, but she smiled as if she could hear her.

JoAnne said, "Do you want to sing, Susie? How about this song—'Pack up all my cares and woe, here I go, swinging low. Bye, bye, blackbird.'" There was no reaction from Susan, so JoAnne added, "Come on, Susie, *sing!*"

"Ow-w-w-w."

"Mumsie, remember how Grandpa used to play the banjo every Sunday afternoon when you were growing up? Grandma Dorothy and you and all of you kids would sing?"

Susan's eyes darted around the room. She did not look like she was taking this in.

JoAnne jumped in: "Dad would sit in his big easy chair, and sometimes there was a fire. The wood always crackled, and it smelled so good. Remember? Maybe Mom would have fixed eggs and potatoes and bacon for breakfast. It tasted so good."

Lily smiled, remembering old photos of her mother as a girl, sitting in her family's living room— floral drapes, gray carpet, a green sectional couch. She'd heard that Grandpa Joe didn't really play well but that his whole family was musical. His uncle had been a banjo maker in Charleston, West Virginia, where he lived.

Lily noticed then that her mother was starting to slump again. Lily's own shoulders were so tight they ached. She was tempted to stop her efforts, but she gave herself a little pep talk: "Keep trying, Lil. Don't give up!"

Lily reached over and adjusted the pillows behind Susan's back. "Come on, Mom," she said. "Sit up a little. Let's sing one of your favorites, 'Bye Bye Blackbird.'" She looked at JoAnne, "Ready?"

"Here we go, sister Sue."

Together, they sang, "Pack up all my cares and woe, here I go, swingin' low. . ."

Susan turned her head to look at them.

Lily said, "Come on, Mom. You know the words: '. . . Bye bye, blackbird.'"

Then, once again Lily and JoAnne were belting out the words together: "Where somebody waits for me, sugar's. . ."

Susan's voice piped in, ". . . sweet, so is she."

The other two women stopped singing. With big eyes, Lily asked her aunt: "Did Mom just say the right words?"

For a moment JoAnne was silent. Susan had been at death's door, and now she was filling in verses for old songs. Was this for real? Finally, JoAnne said, "Let's keep singing."

Lily sang, "No one here can love or. . ."

". . .understand me," Susan croaked.

"Aunt Boo Boo, this is amazing," Lily whispered.

"Great, Susie," JoAnne said. "Let's keep singing."

"Oh, what hard luck stories they all. . .," Lily paused. How did it go?

". . .hand me," Susan said.

"Make my bed," Lily sang on, "and light the light, I'll arrive late tonight."

Again, Susan knew it: "…Blackbird, bye bye."

Lily was so excited she felt like leaping into the air. JoAnne had tears in her eyes. The three of them sang together until Susan was tired.

◆　◆　◆

That evening JoAnne and Lily grabbed a quick dinner in the hospital cafeteria.

Lily was really excited about their singing session. "I think Mom did really well, don't you? That's more words than I've heard from her since she got sick."

"When we were singing those old songs with Susie, I felt like Mom and Dad were really with us," JoAnne said, smiling wistfully. "And Granny and Grampa Smith, too," she added, referring to Lily's great-grandparents. "Music was such a part of our growing up. Grampa Smith was so good at the banjo. Uncle Frank played the accordion and Aunt Vada, the piano. Lots of Sundays the whole family would get together play music and sing."

"I could feel them, too," Lily said, stretching her long legs. "It seemed like they were all standing around the bed, listening to those old songs."

"All rooting for Susie Q."

"All rooting for Mom."

◆　◆　◆

The next morning Lily sat in a chair next to her mom's bed twisting her hair around and around her index finger. Her stomach was on fire from too much coffee and from the hollow feeling of fear she was carrying for her mother's life. Lily stood up and started pacing. When were they coming for the damn MRI? It was so damned difficult not knowing what was wrong with Mom.

Then her mother sat bolt upright in her bed and stared across the room.

Lily stopped pacing and stared. What was this?

In a monotone, Susan said, "August 20. Susan Bruzas. Sixty-seven years old. August 26, 1947. Doctor H. Nurse: Sharon. Virginia Mason."

Lily could see that this was word-for-word what was written on the information board. "Mom!" she said. "Are you reading that? I didn't even know you could still read?"

Susan looked at her daughter blankly and curled up again in a fetal ball on the bed.

"Mom! Mom!" Lily said, reaching out and touching her mother's arm. "Are you back with us?" She felt tears gathering in her throat. This was an emotional roller coaster.

Just then an attendant came into the room with a gurney to take her mother for the MRI. "Ready?" he asked Lily.

"Okay," she said, "let's go for it."

Lily walked, with her hand resting on her mom's shoulder as the attendant wheeled the gurney out of the room and onto the hospital's busy seventh floor. Lily started humming "Side by Side," hoping the familiar tune would soothe her mother. They walked into the large elevator, and the doors closed.

Susan suddenly yelled, "JoAnne! JoAnne! Scared! Scared!"

"Hey, hey, hey, Mumsie," Lily crooned. "Sh-h-h, it's okay. It's okay."

Then, to the attendant, Lily said, "Wow, I don't know where that came from. Those are new words. How are we going to get an MRI if she's already this agitated?"

The elevator opened in what looked like the basement. They turned right down a long dimly lit hall to the radiology department. Lily watched as her mother was lifted onto a long plastic table and prepared for the MRI.

"You'll be okay, Mom. I'm right here."

"I think she'll be fine," the technician said. "She almost seems to be sleeping."

Chapter 11

SUSAN: COMING BACK

I felt like I had been completely absent. It was like coming out of anesthesia. It was as if I was emerging from a big blank. A void. I was waking up. And what I woke up to was hearing someone say, "She's sleeping." I knew they were talking about me.

Was I sleeping? No. I knew I wasn't sleeping.

Looking back on this now, I can see that I was at a turning point. I had to decide whether I would continue on the trajectory I'd been on, one that was headed straight for death or into a life in which I might not be fully conscious, in which I wouldn't be "me" anymore. Or would I decide to come back into the joyous, often underappreciated life I'd been living?

Which was it going to be?

The astute reader will notice that I am once again telling my own story. For the last few chapters, I couldn't write in the first person because I wasn't aware of what was happening *while* it was happening.

Now, we come again to scenes for which I *was* conscious, for which I was mentally present. Fortunately, this continues for the rest of the book—though there were some glitches that we will need to explore.

My very first thought was, *Where am I?* I knew it was someplace dark. Everything looked black.

I seemed to be sitting on a hard-back chair in an amphitheater. I looked around, wondering, *Is there anyone here to help me?*

I looked down to the front of the room and saw a group of people standing on a brightly lit stage. They were shaking their fists at each other. They seemed angry. They were yelling. I could see their faces contort and their lips move—though no sound was coming from anyone's mouth. I thought, *Why is this happening?* Once again, I thought, *Where am I?*

At that point, I started yelling, too. Everything seemed meaningless. I could sense that I had worked so hard in my life, and now it seemed to be for nothing. I felt terrified. . . desperate. I knew I was close to exploding into tiny particles, which would then be sucked into oblivion.

Then I saw her: a young woman standing on the stage. She looked so familiar. She had long chestnut-colored hair and a long, lean body. She was shouting and shaking her fist along with everyone else.

It went through my mind: *I think I know her. . . Oh my goodness! That's Lily!*

The moment I recognized Lily, relief and joy flooded through me. I knew then who I was.

I was Lily's mother!

I began to smile—a smile that started on my face and spread, gradually, throughout my entire being. Before long, my heart was filled with love.

I opened my eyes—this time, my physical eyes—and looked straight up into a glaring light. I was lying flat on my back on a narrow, thin pad on top of a table. I lifted up my head, my chin at a slight angle, and I looked down the length of my body to where three people were standing just on the other side of my feet. These three people were all watching me intently. I blinked several times, and my eyes focused on one face that seemed familiar. It was Lily; her sparkling eyes were wide, and she was looking at me in amazement.

"Hi, Lily," I said.

I heard cheering then and joyous laughter. People started clapping. I knew I was safe. I was with my sweet daughter, and she was grinning at me. She was obviously overjoyed.

She said, "Mom, you're awake, and you know who I am!"

Everyone started talking at once. I heard someone say that they should do the MRI later.

"I agree," Lily said. "I want Dr. H to see this."

In a few minutes I'd been lifted onto a softer mattress, one on wheels, and someone propelled me down the hall with Lily walking beside me.

I tried to tell her what had just been happening for me. "I had an amazing dream," I said. "Well, no, not a dream. . . but a. . . Well, you must know—you were there. You were in it. . .yelling and stuff. Everyone seemed so scared."

"Uh-huh," Lily said.

I could see that she didn't understand, and I really, really wanted her to know that she was the one who had brought me back.

"There were shouts, blazing. . . No, no. Bam! I was afraid of bam. But you. . . love. I was so happy to see you."

"I'm happy to see you too, Mom," Lily said, her lip quivering.

"Oh, it's okay, Sweetie." I longed to tell Lily about my experience in the inky black auditorium and my terror of not knowing who I was until I recognized her. I wanted her to know that it was her love that had brought me back. But for now, it was enough to feel her comforting presence walking beside me.

As we rolled down the corridor, we passed two familiar-looking women sitting on a bench by a doorway. They looked at me with surprise and delight. I smiled and gave them a little wave.

We rolled into a room—probably my room—and after I was settled into the bed, a man in a white jacket with a stethoscope around his neck came in. Lily welcomed him with a few excited words, and for a moment they hugged.

They must really like each other, I thought.

This man walked over to me then, extending his hand to take mine. "Well, hello," he said. "Welcome back." He had a nice smile, dark curly hair, and warm blue eyes.

"Hi," I said.

"Can you tell me what your name is?"

"Susan Bruzas."

"Good. And how old are you?"

"Uh." For a moment, I wasn't sure. Then I remembered. "Sixty-seven." I could feel my heart beating faster. Would I be able to do this? I look at Lily for reassurance.

She said, "You're doing great, Mom."

"Who is *this*?" the doctor said, pointing to Lily.

That, I knew. "It's Lily."

She giggled.

"And she's your...."

"She's my daughter," I said, grinning at her.

"You're doing great," the nice doctor said.

But just the fact that he was asking me questions made me worry. What if I couldn't pass his test?

"One more question."

"Okay."

"Where are you?"

I looked around the room for a few seconds. I said, "I don't think I know." I paused, and added, "I'm in a room. At a. . .hospital?"

"Good job, Mom," Lily says, her eyes twinkling.

The doctor stayed for a while. He gave me more tests, but he didn't ask any more questions. He told me to follow the beam from his tiny flashlight as he moved it around the room, and he pricked the bottoms of my feet with pins and made sure that I was able to feel them.

Some other doctors came in. They all stared at me and talked to Lily and to each other. They were so happy. It was like they were having a party or something. Mary Lou came in, and she stood next to me, talking. I couldn't quite hear what she was saying, but her voice sounded like a tinkling brook. Then I saw JoAnne. JoAnne? How could that be? She seemed to be celebrating with everyone else.

I was just glad to be back. I was glad not to be in that terrible black place anymore. I kept my eyes open as long as I could. I drifted off to sleep with Lily holding my hand.

♦ ♦ ♦

"Mom, don't do that again," Lily said, her eyes piercing mine.

I studied her, trying to decipher what she meant. Her lips were turned downward into an angry frown.

"Do what?" I asked.

Just a short time ago—how long ago had it been?—everyone had been so excited that I was awake and talking. Now, I was in trouble, and I didn't know why.

Lily glanced at a woman nearby who was dressed in blue scrubs with a bunny pattern. Who was she, I wondered. The woman had a clipboard in her hand, and she looked official.

My daughter turned back to me and said, "Don't pull out your food tube." She was speaking firmly and with great emphasis. "You need your food tube, Mom, and if you pull it out again, they're going to have to restrain you again."

I noticed that Lily's voice wavered a little. She wasn't mad at me; she was afraid for me.

The bunny lady stepped in then. "Susan, the food tube is vital," she said. "If you don't get sufficient nutrition, it will lead to loss of weight and strength. We don't want that to happen, do we?"

Was it that thing in my nose they were talking about? I wanted to say something to them. A lot of words were floating through my mind, and finally I grabbed one. I said, "Nose."

Lily picked up on it. "You don't like the tube in your nose—is that it?"

"No." I wanted to tell her that my nose tingled and burned. What I said was, "Pain. Ow!"

"Mumsie, you've *got* to leave it in so you can keep getting better."

"If the nasogastric tube doesn't work," bunny lady said, "we might have to go with a gastrostomy tube that's surgically placed through the abdominal wall." She was talking to me as if I were five years old.

Lily just looked worried. I did what I could to reassure her.

I said, "Okay, Sweetie. It's okay. I'll be all right."

Her shoulders relaxed, and she smiled.

Feeling more at ease, I drifted off to sleep.

◆ ◆ ◆

I opened my eyes. No one was in the room. Where had Lily gone?

I looked outside. The sun had just set, leaving a luscious peach-colored sky. A nurse came in and put a bag of yellowish fluid on my IV stand. My mouth suddenly tasted like iron, and I shifted around in bed.

As if reading my mind, the nurse said, "You need this food to give you energy."

Was it this "food" that was hurting my nose? Why wouldn't these people just leave me alone! There was an endless array of people coming and going, sticking my finger with sharp needles, clutching my arm with blood pressure cuffs, removing blood from my system one vial at a time. The sky grew dark, and the hospital quieted. Still no Lily.

I fell asleep.

A while later something woke me. My room was dark except for a parking lot light that was reflecting off the puddles left by a recent rain.

Huh? I sat up and looked around, amazed. I'd never been able to see a parking lot from my room before. What was happening?

Where was I? Had they moved me to a new room? Something must have happened because I appeared to be sitting in the back seat of an old car in the middle of an empty parking lot.

What?

Chapter 12

HOW DID I END UP IN THE FRED MEYERS PARKING LOT?

I attempted to analyze my surroundings. From what I could see, I was, indeed, in the back seat of a car. It reminded me of Jo-Anne's old '53 Chevy in which I had learned how to drive. At a certain point, I practiced driving that car every weekend. I puttered in large circles around the huge empty parking lot at our high school and, eventually, I white knuckled the six blocks home.

The car had grey upholstered seats and rubber floor mats. The dashboard held a large round speedometer with smaller gauges next to it for gasoline, temperature, and air pressure. Beside the gauges, the name Chevrolet was written in stylish silver letters.

I peered out the window. Puddles on the asphalt reflected the light from the front of what seemed to be an empty superstore. It looked like I was in a Fred Meyer's parking lot along with a couple of deserted cars.

Did the hospital have rooms at Fred Meyer. Perhaps so.

I could see that it was inky black in the back seat. I held my hands up in front of me. They looked very white. I looked closer and saw that I was wearing white mittens. The mittens were tied to my wrists and made of some material that scratched my hands, almost like tiny pieces of glass. I wriggled my fingers—trapped and sweaty in these mittens. I wanted my hands to be free. I couldn't seem to manage that, however, and there was no button to call the nurse for help. I tried to take off one mitten with the other hand, but my fingers just slid around inside the scratchy fabric. Tugging at a mitten with my teeth was also hopeless. I couldn't even scratch my nose.

No one was anywhere around. It was just me in an old Chevy in the Fred Meyer parking lot.

I finally fell asleep.

When I opened my eyes sometime later, it was still dark. The parking lot was uninhabited. My heart began to beat faster, and I shifted around trying to get comfortable. Then I remembered what I used to do when I was a child and I'd wake up in the middle of the night. The whole world would seem to be sleeping. Sometimes my stomach was upset, but I was afraid I'd be in trouble if I called for my mom and woke up my dad. If that happened, Dad would yell, "Go back to sleep!" So, lying there on my own, I'd stare into the blackness and hope to hear a car driving on the highway. That sound would reassure me that someone else in the world was awake. I kept repeating this one thought: *If I can just make myself go back to sleep until morning, everything will be all right.*

So, using my childhood strategy now, I closed my eyes and made myself go back to sleep.

◆　◆　◆

The next morning, I awoke to the sound of two women talking. Little by little I opened my eyes. I was back in my regular hospital bed in the same room I'd been in the day before. A soft sheet and blanket were covering me, and morning sunlight was pouring in through the windows. I'd made it!

My pretty dark-haired little sister, Nadine, was sitting next to me, talking to a young woman in blue scrubs. They didn't know I was awake.

"She's still having processing problems," the woman was saying. "Olivia—that's the other speech pathologist—and I will keep working on that, and we should see improvement, if not a complete recovery.

"Nadine," I said. I was so happy to see my little sister.

"Susie," she said, smiling at me. "I'm so happy you're awake."

"Guess what, you guys?" I asked them both. "This hospital has rooms in the Fred Meyer parking lot."

"Oka-a-ay," Nadine said, her eyes widening. She glanced sideways at the woman whose eyebrows went up a bit.

"Really, they do! That's where I spent the night." I noticed that they didn't seem to believe me. I was really happy to be back in my warm and friendly room. Even though the place had changed, I was still wearing the same pair of mittens.

Later, when I was alone, I managed to take the mittens off, using my teeth. I hid my hands under the blanket and wiggled my fingers. I was finally free.

Before very long, a nursing assistant who had come in to do something noticed my naked hands.

"What did you do?" he asked as he pulled the sheet back. "Why you little. . ."

He was big, male, and muscular, and I felt intimidated. "Please. . .please. . .please," I kept saying. I felt like a little girl who'd gotten into trouble for mischief.

Ignoring me, he tied the mittens back on my hands.

Hours passed before he returned. "Are you going to be a good girl now?" he asked. He wasn't smiling.

I looked at him, puzzled.

"I'll take off the mittens if you agree to stop yanking out the food tube!"

I had no idea what he was talking about, but I was afraid of him. I would have promised anything to get rid of those horrible mittens. Besides I knew I was a "good girl" and whatever I had done wrong, I wouldn't do again.

I bobbed my head up and down, and he finally took the mittens off.

♦   ♦   ♦

Later that morning Lily came and pulled a chair next to my bed. She picked up one of my hands. "I see the mittens are gone," she said smiling.

"Yeah, that mean man took them off."

"The mittens were better than the restraints they put you in. That was awful. You just about went crazy."

"Restraints?" I asked. I was confused. I didn't remember any restraints.

"Never mind, Mumsie. That was last night." She patted my hand. "It's a new day, and the sun is shining. Everything is going to be all right."

I never spent another night in the back seat of an old Chevy, but I was to find myself in many more mysterious circumstances in the hospital.

Chapter 13

LUNCH IN THE CLASSY HOSPITAL RESTAURANT

"Lily. Lily."

She didn't answer and instead looked out the dining room windows. I could hardly blame her. We were sitting in the hospital's capacious restaurant with a spectacular view of Puget Sound. A breeze danced over the icy blue waters and reflected the sparkling light of the sun.

"Lily, I want to go home. Please take me home."

"Mom," she said with a sigh, "you are in no way ready to go home."

"Then give me the keys. I'll drive myself home!"

"I've told you," she sputtered. "You cannot leave the hospital. You can't even walk let alone drive!"

I longed for my sweet white house sitting above its wide street. The neighborhood was so quiet, and I loved the green lawn in front and rockery surrounding it.

I tried to put that into words: "My house. . .so white pretty with the. . .rockery. You know." I seemed to run out of air. These days I couldn't make my breath last.

Lily's eyebrows came together as if she were puzzled. "Rockery? There's no rockery." She shook her head and looked away.

I knew I was annoying her, but Lily was my lifeline to get out of the hospital, and I felt I had to work fast. I had a sinking feeling that she was leaving in a few days.

"Please, Lily. Please." I was begging now, and I started folding and refolding the white cloth napkin.

"Mom, for God's sake."

"Then the train. I love the train. So beautiful to sleep like in Europe. Let's go to Europe."

She mumbled something I couldn't hear.

I looked around the restaurant. People were talking quietly and eating their lunches. Waiters were walking from table to table, pouring coffee into china cups.

"Can I get some coffee?" I asked one of the waiters.

Lily spoke up: "Did you just ask the nurse for coffee? Mom, you can't even have water yet."

"But it smells so good." I sighed.

Lily scooted her chair back and stood up from the table. "I have to use the restroom."

The next thing I knew, Nadine was at the table. I guess lunch was still being served. Then two men with white jackets and name tags appeared.

I recognized the doctor with the kind blue eyes. He visited me every day. I thought of him as Dr. H.

"Hi," I said to him. "This is my sister, Nadine."

He introduced the man beside him. I didn't catch his name. His eyes scrutinized me. I didn't know what to say.

"Do you have any questions?" my nice doctor asked Nadine.

"Well, I was wondering about. . ."

I couldn't understand the rest of what she asked, but both men became very engaged. I was so proud of how intelligent my little sister was.

After the doctors left, Nadine looked at her watch and said, "I've got to go meet Diane for lunch. She's coming over from Bainbridge Island."

Lunch? Didn't she want lunch here in this spectacular restaurant? Why would she have lunch somewhere else? It was all very strange.

Time seemed to warp and bend. One minute I was in the restaurant with sunlight streaming in the window, and in the next, I was back in my room. Night had crept in with a cushioned quiet, interrupted only by people poking my fingers and changing my IV bags.

Then one morning I was all alone. An inchoate ache pulsed in my heart. I was aware of missing someone.

Mary Lou and JoAnne came into the room. I looked past them, expecting another person to come in as well.

I asked "Where's. . .?"

JoAnne sat next to me on my bed. "Let's sing, Susie."

I searched her eyes. She was trying to distract me.

"I know," I said. "Lily went home."

"Yes, Susan," Mary Lou said. "She had to go back to work. But she will call you soon."

"She left me. She was supposed to. . ." I couldn't get the rest out. I was tired and sad.

Why hadn't Lily taken me with her? I just wanted to go home.

♦ ♦ ♦

Dr. H hadn't been by to see me this morning, so I decided it was a good time to practice answering the questions he always asked. I knew all of the answers except what hospital I was in. Then I discovered all of the information I needed was written on the white board next to the doorway. All I had to do was memorize it.

"My name is Susan Bruzas," I read aloud. "I'm sixty-seven years old. I was born August 26, 1947, and I'm in Virginia Mason Hospital." If I could just remember the name of this place. "Virginia Mason. Virginia Mason. Virginia Mason."

Feeling a little hot, I threw off my sheet and blanket. Wasn't the AC working in this room?

Some women from the meditation center came in. They brought me colorful bouquets of flowers, which they put in the bay window.

I was so happy to have these great people come to visit me in this large, lovely hospital room in a Victorian house. There was a plush Persian carpet on the floor, and silk curtains hanging in the window. A soft light showed off the impressionistic art that was hanging on the walls.

More and more people came in my room, and I began calling out their names,

"Susan! Tootsie and Barb! Linda, you're here!" I was thrilled that all these people had come to see me. As they talked to me and to one another, still more people came in. Pretty soon people filled my big round room in my Victorian house.

I started to feel overwhelmed and prickly hot. This was a lot of people. Bright colors flashed in front of me: red, orange, purple, yellow all swirled in a kaleidoscope pattern. I was tired. I closed my eyes.

It was too much. I told myself I was going to have to sneak off. In my beleaguered mind, we were now on a train, and I crept away down the passageway until I found a warm comfortable berth with a golden night light. Here, I would hide away and sleep while the train took me home.

"Oh-h-h," one of my visitors said, leaning down toward my face. "Susan went to sleep."

Ha-ha. I got away.

♦ ♦ ♦

I woke up sometime later. Bright lights were shining in my face. My body ached. and the bed felt like it was tipping from side to side.

"Her temp. is 38.8," a woman's voice said. "Let's page the doc and get an x-ray scheduled so we can look at her lungs."

How high was 38.8? I had no idea. Was that why I felt like I was on fire? I also felt like I was rocking in a rowboat. What was happening to me?

Chapter 14

WHAT IF I FLUNK THIS TEST?

Swirling green coolness brushed my face, refreshing as a soft breeze. A gentle rain shower fell around me, sounding like the ringing of two tiny bells. The purity of the bells transformed into two familiar women's voices. The indistinct sounds morphed into words that consoled and soothed me.

"Her sister said her temperature was high, and for a while they were really worried. They thought she could have pneumonia. But her lungs were clear, so they brought her fever down with Tylenol or something like that. She's on antibiotics now."

"What caused it, do you know?"

"A urinary tract infection. Probably from her catheter. It's been in her forever."

"Poor honey. She's suffered so much."

"At least it's not cancer!"

Was that me they were talking about? I listened intently for a few more seconds, but the voices were quiet. I opened my eyes to morning light and the faces of two of my dear friends, Val and Jenny. With them, it was never just Val or just Jenny. They were always together, friends forever.

We had all worked as speech pathologists. We started getting together after Jenny told us that her birthday wasn't the same after her mom's death. So, from that year on, we made a big deal out of all of our birthdays in relation to the time of the year: a Christmas event for Jenny, a visit to the tulip fields for Val in the spring, and dining outside on a deck over Puget Sound for my summer birthday. The rest of the year we would call for "a Starbucks" when we needed to talk, mostly about the (sometimes harrowing!) path of being a mother.

Seeing Val and Jenny, I just knew everything was going to be okay. I grinned at them.

◆　◆　◆

"Hi Susie Q," Val said, pulling her chair closer to my bed. "How're you doing? Apparently last night you had quite a fever."

Had something been wrong with me last night? I didn't know, so I didn't know what to say.

"Do you need anything," Jenny asked me. "How about some water?"

I beamed. My tongue was sticking to the top of my mouth, and I had a dry throat. "Thirsty," I croaked. Why did my voice sound like that?

Val stood up. "I don't see any water," she said. "Let me see if I can find a nurse."

Just then a young woman with a clipboard came in the room. "Good morning," she said. "I'm Cheryl, the speech and language pathologist assigned to Susan. Are you family?"

Val and Jenny both laughed a little. We were like family. They told her that they were my friends, that we were all speech pathologists, and that they'd worked with me for thirty years in the Northshore School District.

The speech therapist's shoulders hunched a little, and her voice became smaller. She looked scared. I wondered why?

"Oh, um, nice to meet you. I'm actually here to do some informal assessments."

"I see," Jenny said. "Susan spoke the word 'thirsty' when she woke up a minute ago? Can she have some water before she starts?

It might be better for her answering questions, don't you think?" Then she asked, "Do you mind if we stay? We'll be quiet."

"Now, now, now," I giggled. Val and I had teased her more than once about asking so many questions. Jenny's husband had made a half-facetious rule that she was limited to two questions per conversation.

"She's not cleared for any water because there's still a danger of aspiration of fluids into the lungs. But she can use these sponge swabs."

She reached into her pocket and pulled out a swab and unwrapped it. Dipping the sponge in water she put it in my mouth and slid it around.

"Mmmm," I hummed. It felt so good.

"I'll ask someone to bring you more, and you can moisten your mouth by yourself, okay?"

"Okay, but want food. I hate, hate, hate this yellow stuff," I said, pointing at the mustard-colored solution that was hanging from a pole in an IV bag.

"Not until you can swallow better, Susan. Is it all right if your friends stay while I ask you some questions?"

I looked at them and warmth spread through me like a nice cup of tea. My friends were as strong as lions. Of course, I wanted them there.

"Yeah," I said.

They backed up a bit to make room for Cheryl. She sat down by my bed and picked up her clipboard.

"All right, Susan, I'm going to say some words, and I want you to repeat them back to me. Okay?"

"Okay."

"Here we go. Ready? Please, pleasing, pleasingly."

"Please, pleasing, pleasing."

She crossed something off.

"Hope, hoping, hopefully."

"Hope, hopping. . .oh-h-h-h-h." My throat started to get dry and tight again.

"You're doing fine," she said, her eyes softening.

She gave me some more words then, and my head started to swim. Every time I spoke, I sounded like a frog. Why did my voice sound like gravel? And why did I keep running out of breath?

Cheryl said, "Let's try something else."

"Are you going to give her some receptive language items?" Jenny asked, pushing her hair behind her ear.

"One more task, then I will." Then, to me, "Okay, Susan, now I am going to have to repeat as many words as you can in a certain group? For instance, I might say, 'Tell me all the names of fruit that you can.' You could say banana, cherries… and what else could you say?"

"Um, apple, grapes?"

"Yes, that's the idea."

Was she going to get mad at me if I flunked this test?

She took out a stopwatch. Oh no, this was *timed*! I bit my lip hard. I knew I wasn't going to be able to get words out fast. I felt like someone had just shoved me onto a stage and told me to dance. But there was an audience watching, and I couldn't remember the steps!

"You'll be fine, Susie," Val said.

I took a deep breath.

"Okay? Ready? Tell me all of the containers you can think of in one minute. Go!"

"Uh. . . uh. . . box, bed. . .No, that's not right. Bag, potato. . . I mean pot. . ." I looked around the room for ideas.

Val moved her eyes down to her lap, at me, then down to her lap again.

I got it then; she had a water bottle on her lap.

"Bottle," I yelled.

"Good!" Cheryl said, clicking her stopwatch. "Time's up."

"Oh no," I said with a grimace, my face hot with embarrassment. I just knew I had flunked.

"You did good, Susie Q," Jenny said.

Cheryl squeezed my arm and moved on to reading me little stories and asking me questions about them, things like "What time did Brenda go shopping?" and "What did she buy?"

It seemed to me that I bombed that, too. I was frustrated. I couldn't remember the words.

My friends were also taking note, but in a different way. Val asked, "Why is her voice so hoarse?"

Cheryl didn't know, but she made a note. "I'll see if we can get that checked out," she said.

◆　◆　◆

When my interrogator finally left, Jenny pushed the call button and asked, "Could we get some oral swabs for Susan?"

That would help, certainly.

Trying to cheer me up, Val asked me if I'd heard from Alena. I couldn't remember, but then I asked for my phone.

"Your cell phone?" Jenny asked.

I nodded, yes.

They started searching, moving tissue boxes, get-well cards, bedsheets. . . Finally, the phone turned up, plugged into an outlet in the corner of the room to recharge.

"I'm calling Rowan," I said.

"You're calling Rowan?" Jenny asked, looking dubious.

"Yes, calling my grandson."

"What's your password?" Val asked.

I put my hand out, took the phone from her, and typed in the password. That's one thing I do know, passwords!

Then I found Alena's number under "favorites" and pressed it.

I listened to the phone ring on the other side of the call. When I heard Alena's voice in her recorded message, an ache filled my heart. I missed her so much. I wished she was here at the hospital.

After the message ended, I spoke into the phone: "Hi Alena? For Rowan. Meemaw here at, talking. So, want to see voice to you. You're at a. . . a, . . a room building? I lots of tests. Boring. Miss you. Okay? Love you." I clicked off.

Jenny and Val looked at each other and smiled.

"You did it, Susan," Jenny said. "You knew exactly what to do."

"Yeah, good job, Susie."

"I know."

A lady dressed in blue scrubs brought in some oral swabs and Val dipped them in water and handed me one.

I put one in my mouth and sucked. It tasted so good.

"Pretty soon we'll bring you a nice warm mocha," Val said.

A memory of sitting at a Starbucks flashed through my mind. Steam rising from a hot mocha, a sampling of chocolate chip cookies and pumpkin bread on a couple of napkins between us. I'm talking rapidly, gesturing exuberantly with my hands and arms. Val and Jenny are laughing.

I blinked. There was no mocha or plate of cookies, just this mushy cotton swab to suck. Sadness slid through me like thick mud.

"Yeah," I said, managing a smile. "Nice." It had been nice.

Chapter 15

ABANDONED IN
THE WAREHOUSE

Time went by like old vacation slides being projected onto a screen. Morning with bright sunbeams coming in the window. *Click.* Evening with softening light and sound. *Click.* Middle of the night and a quiet person checking my pulse and IV bags. *Click.* Morning again. . .

"Now, we need to get you up in the chair, Mrs. Bruzas."

There was always somebody bugging me. And why was this woman calling me Mrs. Bruzas? I've probably been divorced longer than she's been alive.

But I didn't want to hurt her feelings, and I couldn't get that many words together anyway. What I meant to say was, "Just leave me in bed. I'm tired."

I don't think she heard me. She pulled the nice warm bedding back.

"Cold," I said.

"Come on, let's sit up," she said. "You can swing your legs over to the side. Just slide them over. Here we go."

I wanted her to stop talking to me like I was a little kid. But it occurred to me that I might be acting like a little kid. So, I sat up.

"Now swing your legs so they're hanging over the edge."

"What?"

"Here, like this." She picked up my legs and started moving them to the side of the bed. "Now, you try."

"My legs feel like they weigh two tons."

"I know. You've said that, but you have to try."

I realized I *had* said that over and over, and I'd done that because my legs *did* feel like they weighed a lot. But then I tried, and in a few moments my feet were dangling over the side of the bed, just like she'd wanted them to.

"Now, scootch your bottom toward the edge of the bed."

I leaned back on my arms and pushed and managed to slide my butt forward little by little.

"Now, I'm going to cinch this belt around you. Then I'll help you stand up, turn a little, and get you safe and snug in your chair."

I looked at my bed longingly. I just wanted to sleep.

Nevertheless, between the two of us I ended up sitting in the chair.

"Okay, good. Now you can look out the window if you want. And I will be back in a little while."

I felt my chest tightening. I was terrified of being stuck in the chair, exhausted and alone.

I just knew that other patients would distract her. She was going to take a long time to get back to me. I just knew it!

"Wait," I told her. "Don't leave. Don't leave me here!"

"Don't worry. You'll be fine Mrs. Bruzas."

"Susan!" I put a lot of energy into conveying that name.

"Okay. Susan. I will be back in a few minutes to check on you."

"Oh, all right," I said, feeling depleted. Feeling left. Feeling alone.

After a while I looked around my room. They were always moving me. Usually, it was in the middle of the night. I'd wake up, and I'd be somewhere else. I'd been in this room before, though. It was the UW professor's office.

It was nice of this professor to let me use his room. He must be on summer break.

I looked out the window at the other campus buildings. The dormitory windows were winking in the sunlight. I squinted my eyes to try and spot students, but all I could see was the sun reflecting back. It seemed very quiet for a campus, even for summer vacation.

"Well, hello. I see they have you sitting up."

"Hi, doctor." It was the nice doctor whose name started with an H. I could never remember it. He had such kind eyes. "Yep, they said it would be good for me."

"And how are you feeling?"

"I'm exhausted."

"You've been through a lot," he said in a gentle voice.

"And I'm sick of this food tube. It tastes like iron. And I'm hungry."

"I see." He made a note on my chart.

He moved a chair close to mine and looked at me intently. "The other doctors and I think that you've had viral encephalitis."

"Viral what?"

"Viral encephalitis, which was most likely caused by the medication you were taking for your lupus. It suppressed your system to the point it allowed a virus to get into your brain."

"It let a virus into my brain. Jeez." I pictured little bugs crawling around inside my head.

The doctor went on to explain my white blood cells were not able to do the job of fighting off the virus that got into my system— or had already been hiding in my body, like chicken pox. Now, I had been taken off this medicine that had been keeping down my white blood cells.

"That medication was designed for people who've had organ transplants," the doctor said. "They have to take it."

"So, their bodies don't reject their new organ," I said, interrupting him.

His eyebrows shot up and he smiled, maybe because I was able to understand his explanation. But it felt like I was in a dream. It wasn't really me we were talking about. It was some interesting student that I had on my caseload. Or maybe it was someone on a good episode of House or ER.

Before Dr. H left, he said he'd ask the speech person for another swallowing test to see if I could begin a diet of soft food.

Later that day, Cheryl came in and made me practice swallowing glops of different stuff. I liked the pudding. After it was over, she said I could start drinking liquids and eating soft foods. If I ate enough, they would take away one bag of the iron-tasting yellow glop.

♦　♦　♦

The next morning Mary Lou came in for her visit. She had been here every morning and evening since I'd been in the hospital.

"Guess what!" I told her.

"What?" She put her bag down and sat by my bed.

"I can eat soft foods now."

"Really?"

"And soup. I really miss dal."

"I know, Susan. I miss going out for Indian food with you, too."

I realized that I had no memory of going out for Indian food with anyone. I couldn't even picture being in a restaurant. What I could remember is a wonderful combination of red or yellow lentils with spices.

"No, no, no. I miss dal. Could you bring me some dal?"

"Are you sure it's all right?"

I suspected it wasn't, but I figured I could sneak a little. "Well, it's soft," I said, "and easy to swallow."

"Okay." Mary Lou was going along with me, but her brows were furrowed with worry.

That evening, Mary Lou brought me some dal, which wasn't like I remembered. It was runny and tasted like onions. I tried to eat as much as I could so Mary Lou wouldn't be mad. After she left, I hid the rest under some tissues, hoping a nurse didn't find what might be considered contraband. I snuggled down into bed, put my mantra on my phone and went to sleep.

I woke up at some point in the night, wondering where I was. Had they moved me again?

It was dark and the hospital was quiet. I looked around at the huge room I was in. In the dim light I could see wooden floors and walls. Fear hit my chest like sharp shards of glass. Had they put me in a warehouse?

I pictured a building with many rooms on the waterfront, an old structure with pilings holding it up. I had the terrifying sensation of being small, almost invisible.

Where was everyone? The nurses must be far away.

A wave of nausea went through me. Shivering, I pulled the cover up underneath my chin.

I figured I'd just close my eyes and go to sleep. I told myself, "Go to sleep and everything will be all right."

I tried to sleep, but I tossed and turned. My stomach was roiling, and my mouth tasted like onions. It had sounded so pleasurable to celebrate being able to eat soft food by having some Indian dal soup. How was I supposed to remember that onions upset my stomach? And why didn't someone come now to help me? I rummaged around for the call button, but I couldn't find it.

Was there no one here? It occurred to me that the closest nurse must be at the other end of this warehouse, miles and miles away.

I bit my lip to keep myself from crying. I felt so alone. Everyone was asleep but me—everyone in this hospital, in this city, in this world. What could I do? I was afraid I was going to throw up. I just hate throwing up! What I needed to do is sleep until morning. If I could just make it through the night, I'd be all right.

Finally, I fell asleep.

When I woke up, I could feel that someone or something was in the room with me.

Was it one of those enormous waterfront rats?

I peered into the dark and made out the figure of a nurse standing by my bedside. Finally!

"I feel really sick," I said as he clipped an oximeter on my finger.

"You feel sick?" he repeated, sounding concerned.

"Yeah, I've felt sick all night long. I think I might throw up. Can you give me some Compazine?" I don't know how I remembered the name of that anti-nausea medicine, but I knew that it really worked.

"That's pretty strong," he said. "I'd have to ask the doctor. What's on your diet?"

He looked at the whiteboard, which said I was on soft foods. I wasn't about to tell him I'd eaten dal. I was afraid that he'd yell at me. He left me with a small plastic dish with instructions to throw up in it if I needed. I didn't see him after that.

◆ ◆ ◆

"Susan, can you wake up. Susan, time to open those beautiful eyes. You've been sleeping all morning. Let's get you up."

"Huh? It's morning?" I opened my eyes a little to the bright room and saw a figure in a blue jacket leaning over me.

"Actually, it's almost noon. You've been groaning. Are you in pain?"

"Yes," I said, "I am." It was the speech therapist.

"Can you show me where the pain is?"

"I don't know."

"Is it your stomach? The night nurse said you were nauseated."

"Yeah, I threw up all night long. I want to just rest now."

Someone else came in the room and said, "You need to take your medication, Susan. I have them broken up and in the applesauce like you like."

"What do you mean?"

"You can take a spoonful of the applesauce along with your medication," this person, probably a nurse, said.

"You're not making any sense. Go away and let me sleep." I was starting to feel angry. Why did they talk such gibberish! Why wouldn't they let me sleep!

"Susan, it's really important to take your meds. In fact, one of them will help settle your stomach."

"You're just not making any sense. I'm sorry." I turned on my side and closed my eyes. They talked to each other for a while, and I could understand every word that they said.

"She told the night nurse she'd been vomiting, but there was no evidence that she had," one person said.

"Maybe she just felt sick and didn't actually vomit," the other person said. "She wasn't dehydrated."

Finally, they left, and I went to sleep.

Time coalesced into a series of moments flashing into my awareness—again like the shifting scenes of a slide show.

Click: My arm was encased in a blood pressure cuff. *Wisht-wisht-whisht* it said as it became tighter and tighter around my arm.

Click: The sound of a chair scraping toward my bed. "Let's just sit here for a while and see if she wakes up," whispered someone.

I tried hard to open my eyes, but my lids felt like they were in thick maple syrup.

"Looks like she needs to sleep. Let's visit another time."

Click: "Hi Susan. You've slept all day now, so maybe we can get you up before it's time for dinner."

I opened my eyes and looked around. There was still sunlight in the room, but it had dimmed.

"Come on, let's sit you up."

I felt like she was yanking me around. "You people want me to move in such a hurry!" I said. "I'm not crazy!"

Her eyebrows went up in surprise. I hadn't meant to hurt her feelings. She said some more words to me about sitting up.

"I don't know what you mean. How do I do it?" I felt anxious and confused.

She gave me more directions. Finally, I figured out what she was talking about and, I was able to get up and into the chair. But I was so weary. My body felt heavy and sluggish.

"I don't want to be in the chair," I said. "I told you I was awake all night. What I want to do is go back to bed."

She left me there anyway. I looked around. At least I was out of the warehouse and back in the professor's office.

♦ ♦ ♦

That evening they wanted me to order something from the menu for dinner.

Why would I do that when I'd puked all night? It's like they didn't believe that I was really sick. I wasn't about to tell them that the onions in the dal made me sick. Mary Lou might get in trouble.

So, they hooked me up again to the iron-flavored food supplement.

Oh no! Would I ever get to eat real food again? This had happened because I broke the rules. I was so mad at myself. Now I'd never get out of here.

Chapter 16

MY DEAR, YOU WERE OUT OF THIS WORLD

"I want my birthday cake," I told JoAnne.

"I know, Susie. You've been saying that for days. But you're not allowed to eat regular food yet."

"I don't want this crappy food tube," I said. "I want cake and ice cream."

"I know. I'm sorry," my sister said, sighing. "Look, I brought you some birthday balloons." She started tying them to one of the chairs in the room.

I watched JoAnne at her task. She seemed to be floating in a bubble—maybe because she was happy to be with me. My sister kind of looked like her best friend, Rea, who was always giggly and cheerful. It's just that unlike JoAnne's reddish-brown hair and five-foot-five frame, Rea had white-blonde hair and stood a diminutive five feet.

But why did I keep thinking about Rea? It's JoAnne who was here. Couldn't I just enjoy that my sister was with me to celebrate my sixty-eighth birthday. It occurred to me that I was going to have to try to remember my new age because around here I was constantly being asked how old I am.

I focused on JoAnne then. "The balloon is pretty," I told her.

"I'm just so happy we didn't lose you and that you're around for another birthday!"

"You always find me."

"What do you mean?" she asked, sitting down close to me.

"Remember when I was little and I'd walk in my sleep? I'd open my eyes. It would be pitch black, and I'd yell for help."

"Like when you woke up in our bedroom in the middle of the night, and you didn't know where you were?" JoAnne asked.

"Oh yeah, I remember."

I must have been about eight and JoAnne eleven. We shared the same double bed in a small bedroom with a tan linoleum floor and one narrow wooden closet that was the stuff of nightmares. I had woken up in inky darkness, confused and terrified. I could feel that I was sitting on top of a small space that was solid and smooth.

"Help," I'd whimpered, terrified that I was going to fall off. My heart was hammering hard in my chest. "Help," I said a bit louder.

"Susie, what are you doing?" JoAnne said in a tired, irritated voice.

"I don't know where I am."

"Okay," she said, her voice nearer to me. "You're all right. Just scoot your butt forward."

I scooted.

"Now put your hand out and take hold of the bed frame."

I felt around and grasped the cold brass bedstead.

"Now climb over."

"What? I can't see-e-e-e." I was about to panic, but JoAnne tugged my hand and pulled me up and onto the mattress.

We both laughed at this memory. It was amazing I could actually remember and talk about it.

"Remember I'd asked you if I was okay, and you said, 'You're fine just go back to sleep?'"

"Yeah, and your feet were by my head," JoAnne recalled. "I just wanted you to go back to sleep so I said that.

"Where had I been sitting?"

JoAnne paused for a moment. "Oh, I know," she said. "You must have been walking in your sleep. You somehow got yourself on top of the wooden case that held the old record player that Mom and Dad stored in our bedroom."

That made sense. Then I focused again on my big sister. "You were always rescuing me, JoAnnie. You still do."

"You fought to get better all by yourself, Susie. It's a miracle you're still alive."

I wondered what she meant by that. Of course, I was still alive! After a while JoAnne left the professor's office to go to the bathroom.

I noticed then that I was back in the office. They must have put me back here while I was sleeping. I wondered if JoAnne would see any students wandering by.

When she came back I asked her, "What's out there?"

She looked mystified for a moment. "What's out there?"

"Yeah, what's out there?"

"Well, the restroom is right outside the door. Down the hall is an elevator and across from that is the…you know, the. . ."

"The receptionist area?"

"Well, yes."

In my mind's eye I could see a receptionist greeting the teachers and students, answering questions, and the phones.

JoAnne hadn't mentioned students, so they must all still be on summer break.

We spent the rest of the day together, JoAnne floating up and down in her happy bubble answering phone calls for me and greeting friends that came to wish me a happy birthday.

♦　♦　♦

Days passed with the light from a white-hot sun filling my room. One of my attendants said it was the hottest summer on record. And I'd missed it. I yearned to be swimming in the cool waters of Lake Washington or sitting outside, under an umbrella, eating fish and chips with Val and Jenny. I was still hooked to the food tube, but today the speech pathologist was going to be checking to see if I could go on solid food again.

I awoke late one morning to find Mary Lou sitting quietly beside me. Her presence was always calming. Then a young man with light blue eyes came in and introduced himself as my new SLP.

"Oh good," I said. "I didn't like that other lady. She'd never let me eat food."

"Well, let's see how you do today."

He gave me water, crackers, and some mushy stuff to eat, and he stared at my throat while I swallowed.

"I don't like that mushy stuff," I said, "and I'm not swallowing anymore." I looked at Mary Lou for support.

"You want to eat regular food again, don't you?" she asked.

"Yes, but that tastes so bad I'm not eating it. I'm not a baby."

"If you could eat anything in the world right now, what would it be?" the SLP asked.

"A root beer float!" I'd answered right away.

"Okay, finish this one little exercise, and we'll get you one."

"And I want organic ice cream and good root beer, not a cheap brand. I know because I bought root beer for our center to celebrate our guru's birthday."

"Okay, if you can finish up the swallowing test for me."

"Okay."

I completed the test, and the SLP promised to send a helper to get exactly what I'd ordered.

"Thank you. I can't wait," I exclaimed.

"Meanwhile, you can work with the physical therapist on walking. She's been waiting."

"Oh no. Not that again. I don't want to walk. I want to be in a wheelchair."

"Susan," Mary Lou said, her brows furrowing. "You need to get stronger before you can go home so you can walk up those front stairs, right?"

"Walk?" That seemed a million days away.

"Come on, Susan," the physical therapist said. "Let's get you up. We've got to work up an appetite."

"I have no idea what you mean, but okay."

After much effort, I was finally sitting on the edge of the bed feeling depleted, dizzy, and drenched with sweat.

Why didn't anyone understand how I felt? Mary Lou was my friend! Couldn't she see how impossible this was for me?

The physical therapist certainly couldn't see. "Let's stand up," she said in a cheerful voice, "and get you to grab onto the walker."

"No-o-o-o," I protested.

"Let's walk down the hall to the sunroom, and by the time you get back your root beer float will be here."

God, they were talking to me like I was a baby. Were they going to give me a shiny sticker if I cooperated? But I knew that I'd better not say anything. I might make the physical therapist cry.

After dragging myself halfway down the hall, I refused to go any farther.

"That's it. I want to go back and have my float."

"That's it?"

"Yep."

She finally allowed me to go back to the room, and soon I was drinking a delicious root beer float. Which *was* wonderful.

I asked the SLP, "Can I eat regular food again?"

"We'll start you back on soft food and reduce the food supplement."

"That's a good start, Susan," Mary Lou said.

"Yeah, thanks," I said to the SLP. I really liked him.

♦ ♦ ♦

Later that afternoon the physical therapist came back and tried to get me to stand up again.

"I can't," I said. "I just can't do it."

A nurse was there, too, and she asked me, "What's the matter, Susan?"

I liked this nurse, Sharon. She was kind of tough and ignored my complaints, but she did listen to me, and she seemed competent.

"What do you feel when you try to stand up?"

Finally, someone was asking me how I felt! Somehow, I managed to bring together the right words: "I feel hot, weak, and dizzy!"

The nurse and physical therapist looked at each other in surprise.

"Let's take your blood pressure," Sharon said.

After a minute she said some numbers, and the physical therapist wrote them down.

Then, they both helped me to stand up, I held onto the walker, and Sharon took my blood pressure again. The room started swirling around and little particles of darkness scintillated at the edge of my vision. I half fell back down on the bed.

"Oh, I'm so dizzy."

Sharon said some more blood pressure numbers to the physical therapist.

"Wow, that's quite a drop."

Sharon's eyes narrowed with concern. She said, "Let's page the doc right away."

All that night it seemed like someone was in my room helping me sit and then stand up while they took my blood pressure. It was exhausting, and every time I stood, I felt like I was going to faint. They were so apologetic that I tried to cooperate and not complain.

The next day I told Jenny and Val about my night of interrupted sleep.

"How about we bring you a mocha?" Val asked.

"That would be great. It will be just like Starbucks," I answered, leaning forward with anticipation.

"Okay, and maybe we can have it in the sunroom at the end of the hall."

I nodded although I didn't think I'd ever been down to the end of the hall. I visualized a little room with sun pouring in the two little windows.

A lady in blue scrubs came in and emptied the garbage cans.

"Hi," I said. "How are you?"

She looked up, surprised. "I'm good, thank you."

"I really appreciate how clean you keep the room. You work so hard, coming in here day after day."

"It's nice that you notice," she said with a big smile on her face.

After she left, I watched people walking by and listened to the murmuring of voices and squeaking of carts.

Sharon came in wheeling her computer with her. She didn't say anything to me but started tapping away at her computer. Then she got two IV bags out with something red in it.

"What's that?" I asked.

"RBC units for you: red blood cells to help you feel better."

"Is it my blood?"

"No, but you don't have to worry about that."

"I don't like this one bit."

Ignoring me, she attached the IV bag to the stand and its tube to my PICC line.

Val and Jenny walked into the room talking to each other.

"Sharon, my friends are here. How much longer will this take?"

"More than an hour."

"But I want to have a mocha in the sunroom with them," I said, my voice rising.

Sharon just shook her head.

Without a word, my friends set the drink down and left.

I sighed and leaned back on my pillow. There was nothing I could do but give up. I thought, *I surrender.* The mocha remained untouched, growing cold.

♦ ♦ ♦

They'd moved me again. This time I had a roommate. The last roommate I remembered was an African American lady. I'd whispered to Lily that I was sure she'd been married to a famous rock star like Little Richard. Maybe that's why her television was playing loud rock 'n' roll twenty-four hours a day. Lily had said she thought it was a TV station that played Christian music.

This roomie was on the phone constantly, telling people she'd be home soon and that she was going to take a shower and get packed.

A shower? That sounded wonderful! I hadn't had a shower for eons. I wanted a shower, too.

I buzzed the nurse and asked if I could take a shower.

"Are you sure you're ready?" he asked, looking at the sign above my head—Brain Lesions. Fall Danger.

"I'm not dizzy anymore, and I'm eating regular food, too. I really feel energetic. I've been going to the bathroom by myself, too!"

"Okay," he said. "Let's try it. I'll help you get ready, and I'll sit right outside, in case you need me."

The warm streaming water flowing down my body felt like I had just dived into a warm turquoise inlet on some tropical island. I felt as if I had been camping for weeks and my sweaty, sticky body was finally being cleansed. I stayed in the shower until my energy started to wane. After drying off as well as I could, I pushed the button to call for my attendant.

He was smiling. He asked, "Did that feel good?"

"Heavenly."

I ate an Asian salad for lunch, and then Dr. H came into my room and pulled up a chair.

"You've been doing very well," he told me. "These last five days the improvement has been remarkable. All of your blood tests look good. You're eating solid food well, and those pesky fevers have disappeared."

"I feel really good. I have so much more energy."

"A week ago, we were thinking about long-term care, but now I think a rehabilitation facility is the best setting for you. They can monitor you and help you improve your strength until you're walking steadily with the walker. You might need a little more speech therapy for those cognitive skills also. But I expect you to make a full recovery!"

My heart swelled with excitement and appreciation. I knew the hospitalists were on a two-week rotating schedule, and Dr. H had traded with another doctor so he could spend more time with me.

I thanked this kind doctor for helping me, and for sticking with me.

"Well, you were an interesting case," he said with a smile.

"I guess I was a little out of it at times."

"My dear, you were out of this world, out of this galaxy, out of this universe."

Well, I hadn't felt *that* out of it. But, in fact, this doctor had been present when I'd woken up from the mysterious vision in which I'd felt as if my body was going to disintegrate, and he had heard my garbled explanation of how my love for my daughter was what brought me back.

It doesn't matter. After being in the hospital for so long, I am well enough to finally leave. I wonder where the rehab is. What it will it be like?

Chapter 17

TINY SHIMMERING RAINBOWS

O h my God, I was really, really leaving! Was it still hot out? I peered out the window and saw that the sky was no longer a glaring blue. The sun was hidden behind a bank of gray clouds.

It looked a lot cooler than it had been when I arrived. What time of the year was it now? Late August? September? I wondered what kind of clothes I had with me.

I bit my lip and looked around the room. Then I remembered that Mary Lou had brought some sweats and a T-shirt. I buzzed for someone to come and help me get dressed.

Soon a pleasant dark-haired woman walked into my room. "Can I help you?" she asked.

"Yes, I get to go home. . . Well, not go home but to a rehab place. Anyway, I need to get dressed." I finished on a positive note.

"Oh, that's wonderful," the woman said. "Do you have some clothes to put on?"

I directed her to the paper bag that Mary Lou had brought, and she pulled out my black sports bra and a huge pair of greying white panties.

Wow, those were old—and big! I could feel my face getting warm with embarrassment. But my dressing assistant wasn't as judgmental as I was. Standing on shaky legs, I leaned on her, and together we managed to get the panties on. The bra was more of a struggle.

"Guess I got very saggy while I was here," I said.

We both giggled, and she finally managed to latch the bra in the back. When she was finished, I adjusted the clothes a bit. It felt strange to be so confined by underwear, but the sweatpants felt soft and roomy. I thanked the woman profusely, and then she left.

After lunch another person brought in some boxes and started packing up some of my things. Then he got a call to help someone else.

"That's okay," I told him. "I can call a friend and get them to come."

"Are you sure?"

"Oh, yeah. It's fine."

As I went down the list of friends in my mind, I realized I'd possibly miscalculated. Now that the schools were in session, Val, Jenny, and Mary Lou had all gone back to their jobs. My relatives had all gone home.

Who the heck could come and help me?

Anxiety crept in, making my stomach clench. I took a few breaths and repeated the mantra for a few minutes.

It occurred to me that Mary K might be available. Mary K McCoy was a colleague from my school district. She worked in a school that served children with severe to profound disabilities. When I'd first started, I had little experience working with people at that level, and Mary K had given me the confidence to open myself up and learn as fast as possible. After we'd worked together for a couple of years, she fought a battle with ovarian cancer and won. Ever since, she had been helping cancer survivors get back their physical strength by dragon boating, hiking, and community building.

The question was, would she be home? And if she was, would she be willing to drop everything and come over to help?\

Mary K answered my phone call right away, delighted to hear from me and asking how I was.

"Great!" I told her. "I'm leaving the hospital! I'm being discharged today and going to rehab."

"Oh, that's wonderful. You've done so well."

"I was wondering if you can come over and help me pack up my stuff?"

"Of course. When do you need me?"

"Would right now be okay?"

"Sure. I'll be right there."

In a short time, Mary K walked through the door. She stood five-eight in her stocking feet—the sort of woman my dad used to call "a long, cool drink of water." I think that means a person is refreshing—and Mary K certainly was that for me in this moment.

"Mary K, it's so good to see you," I told her.

"And it's so good to see you. Now what do we need to do here?" And she started right in.

Soon, the two of us had strategized what should go where. It was amazing how many cards, gifts, books, and photos I had in my room. Everyone had been so kind and supportive. Before long, everything was almost done except for a big plastic bag in the back of my closet. Mary K pulled out my blue silk top and crystal necklace.

"Wow," she said, holding up the necklace. "Beautiful! Where are these from?"

It was the blouse and jewelry I had worn so many weeks ago to the Gurupurnima celebration. I could almost feel the warm July night and see the luminous full moon, radiant in the sky, as Ann drove me to the hospital.

"It's what I was wearing at the celebration at my meditation center," I explained.

"It seems so long ago. It was the night I got sick. The necklace is from India. It's actually a *mala*. You use a *mala* by repeating your mantra as you touch each bead."

Sunlight struck the necklace as Mary K held it up. Tiny shimmering rainbows danced on the wall. It was unusually quiet in the room. Rainbows always meant a promise fulfilled to me, or prayers that would be answered. There had been many prayers for my healing, and today I was getting out of the hospital with the hope of a full recovery.

◆　◆　◆

Mary K finished the packing and gave me a farewell hug. Soon after she left, my cell phone rang. It was my sister JoAnne.

I explained that I couldn't talk just then, that I was being transferred to a rehab place, and that the transport was coming any minute now.

"What?" JoAnne said—she was almost shouting, "You're getting out? Where are you going?"

"I. . .um, I don't remember the name. I gotta go, they're coming. Bye."

"Wait," she said, sounding frantic. "What kind of rehab? Are you sure you're ready? I thought you felt really weak?"

"I'm fine, don't worry, bye."

I hung up. I didn't want to have time for phone calls. I wanted my transport to come.

Time went by with no one showing up. I had to eat another high-carb hospital meal with no fresh vegetables. I hoped the new place had better food. Soon, the shadows were growing long, and I began to worry.

Were they ever going to come?

Finally, a nurse came to the door and announced that the ambulance crew was here. A young man and woman came in wheeling a stretcher. They were dressed in tight-fitting black and orange outfits that appeared to be made of Lycra. It reminded me of what high-fashion bike racers might wear. These two looked ready for action.

Was I about to be medevacked in a life flight helicopter? The nurse and I looked at each other, confused.

"I think we ordered the wrong ambulance," the nurse said. "She doesn't need this level of transport," she said.

"Yeah," I agreed. I was going to have to pay for this, and they looked expensive.

The medevac people shrugged and left. Now I had to wait for another simpler and less pricey transport.

Was I going to have to spend another night in the hospital? Would I have to take my clothes off and get into another hospital gown?

I looked around at the room, with my boxes cluttering the floor, and stacks of gloves, tissues, and hand wipes that the hospital for some reason had stored on the shelves and window ledges.

Eventually, a nice young man appeared dressed in ordinary clothes. He helped me get into a wheelchair and pushed me out of the room. As we entered the seventh-floor hall, I was greeted by hospital sounds—a murmur of voices, the creaking of wheelchairs on the move, and an impersonal voice paging a doctor. I was so glad to be leaving all this behind.

"Goodbye," I sang out to the medical staff. "Goodbye, and thanks so much!" I waved like a queen, feeling as happy as if I were in a ticker-tape parade with confetti floating down. Some of the staff gave me a blank look as if to ask, "Now, who is she?" But some smiled and waved. Then they went back to their computers or went off to look after their patients. Maybe they had a room to get ready for a new patient. In my heart I wished them the very best. I had survived, and they were a huge part of saving me. Of course, the prayers offered on my behalf had helped too,

I turned to the man who was wheeling me through the hospital. "What's your name?" I asked him.

"James," he said, smiling.

"Well, thank you, James, for coming out so late. I was beginning to think I wouldn't get to leave today."

"I'm usually on call for any rides someone needs to go home or to rehab, like you."

As we went through the door that took us outside, I breathed in truly fresh air for the first time in weeks.

"Ah, that smells so good. There is nothing like the smell of the air in Seattle—a mixture of the earth and a slight bit of salt from the Salish Sea. And it's so clean! It's just-nectarian."

James smiled and nodded his head. He opened the back of his van, put a ramp down, and wheeled me up. Then he latched the wheelchair in front and back, so I was secure. As we drove away, I was nervous but excited. It was still hard for me to imagine anything out of the reality that I had been living in for so long now. But I sensed that this was a new beginning and a relaxed way of living, sleeping in, visiting friends, and having some good fresh food. I thought it would be a smooth road from rehab to home.

But that was not to be.

Chapter 18

NO WONDER YOUR LEGS ARE SO WEAK

It was growing dark by the time I was wheeled through the front doors of my new home. Rehab was a one-story building with a long row of dimly lit windows looking out on deep green lawn. Just inside the door, in front of a large, curved reception area cluttered with files and desk chairs, a woman stood smiling at me. She was petite and gray-haired.

"Susan? I'm glad to see you," she said. "I'm Sara, and I'm going to get you settled in your new room."

I told her that I was very happy to be there.

I tipped the van driver generously, and, after check-in, Sara pushed my wheelchair down a quiet long hall with light gray carpet and beige walls. Wheeling past a room, I could see an aide tucking a woman into bed and, in another room, a woman getting her blood pressure taken.

"We're in the post-acute section," Sara told me. "This is where we will get you strong enough to go home. I'm an occupational therapist, and I will be working with you along with speech and physical therapists."

I sighed. Not more physical therapy! And why would I need speech therapy? I was talking just fine, and I was eating regular food.

"Here we are," Sara said. "Your new home!" She rolled me into a small room with a single hospital bed, a large fake leather recliner, two small windows, and a bathroom.

"This is nice," I told her. "And it looks like I have no roommate."

"All the rooms in this section are private," Sara said, pulling drawers open and grabbing a blue pullover gown. "You can put this on, and we'll unpack the clothes you brought in these middle drawers so you can reach them. Let's get you situated so you can get into bed since it's almost nine o'clock," she said as she pushed a button to raise the bed.

All of a sudden, I felt a slight stirring in my bowels. Oh no! I needed a toilet right *now*! Could I hold it? I *had* to hold it! I squeezed my bottom, but almost immediately I felt a dampness in my underwear.

"I'm so sorry, but I had a. . .um, a little accident."

Without a word Sara pulled open another drawer, took out padded paper underpants as big as a large diaper, and handed them to me. I felt my face get hot with embarrassment, but her gentle efficiency helped me feel better.

Soon, I was clean and dressed in a comfortable soft blue nightie. Sara said good night, and a nursing aide got me settled. I looked around my dark room, the streetlights illuminating the plants and cards given to me by well-wishers. It was so quiet and peaceful. I switched on my phone and went to sleep listening to my guru singing the mantra.

♦ ♦ ♦

SMASH! SMASH! Chip, chip, tinkle. My eyes flew open.

What was that? Had something broken?

I sat up in bed and listened. There it was again: *SMASH! Chip, chip, chip.* It was coming from the hallway, and it sounded like it was close to my room. The soft sound of the mantra still played as I picked up the phone to check the time.

It was 4:25 a.m.—which seemed too early to be hearing people in the hallways.

Anyway, it was quiet right now, so I decided to lie back down and take some deep calming breaths. After a few minutes I began drifting to sleep. Then my door opened, and a water pitcher was set on my bedside table. I heard the hollow glugging sound of liquid being poured into my glass. I sat up again and took a long drink of cold sweet water. After weeks of feeling parched, this water tasted delicious.

The next thing I knew, early morning sunlight was slanting through the window. I could hear traffic going by outside on the busy street with intermittent honks.

Where was I in the city, anyway? I hadn't noticed on the drive here, and I hadn't asked the driver. Was this residential? If I could get out of bed, I could look out the window and see. But there was no walking for me right now.

A pretty, dark-haired nursing assistant came in my room "Time to get up, honey," she said in a mellifluous voice. She smiled and drew the covers back from my bed.

"No more breakfasts in bed for me," I said.

She just smiled.

Crap! Did this mean that for every meal I had to get up, get dressed, and get down to the dining area? Oh well, maybe I could have a good conversation with other patients.

The assistant pushed me down the long-carpeted hall, chatting with me and saying an occasional "good morning" to other residents. From what I could see, my new home was decorated in a 1970s style: the beige walls were bisected by a wide orange stripe. The air smelled fresh, with no antiseptic hospital aromas greeting my nose.

The dining room held six or seven small round tables. There was a bank of windows that opened to a well-manicured lawn and bright hanging flower baskets. Servers were standing by trays of food and drinks, and I chose some pale-yellow scrambled eggs and orange slices and then was pushed over to a round table with a gray-haired man sitting in a wheelchair.

"Good morning," I said, smiling.

He gave me a blank look.

"It's a lovely day, isn't it?"

He pushed his wheelchair back from the table, turned it at an angle, and tried to get up.

"Whoa," I yelled, reaching my hand out.

Then he tried again and almost fell flat on his face.

"Stop!" someone said. I looked around, and an aide was sprinting across the room to catch him before he fell.

"Okay, okay," the aide said. "You have to be a little patient, Jim. I'm taking you back right now."

No one else came to join me, so I ate the bland-tasting eggs and sliced orange and drank my coffee. A slight assistant with tan skin came and looked at my plate.

"Are you all done?" he asked.

"Um, I think so."

He wrote something down on his clipboard.

"What is this all about?"

"Just writing down how much you're eating, because. . ."

He didn't fill in the reason, but I knew why. It was because I'd refused to eat after I got sick. I never told them why I stopped eating, and after I did, they'd put that horrible food tube in.

I made a promise to myself to eat everything, no matter how bland it was.

I sat sipping my lukewarm coffee, wishing I had someone to talk to. I looked longingly at a group of women talking and laughing at a table near the window. Some of them had walkers by their chairs, and one was in a wheelchair, but they seemed to have normal communication.

"Mrs. McAllister! Oh, Mrs. McAllister," a voice shouted behind me.

I turned and saw a gray-haired woman sitting in her wheelchair in the middle of the room.

No one paid much attention.

"Mrs. McAllister. Hickory dickory dock. The mouse went up the clock," the woman in the wheelchair chanted.

Who was Mrs. McAllister? This woman's nursing assistant? Her kindergarten teacher?

"Mrs. McAllister," she moaned.

"It's okay," I said. "She'll be here soon."

It didn't seem to console this woman one bit as she continued calling for Mrs. McAllister and reciting that insipid nursery rhyme.

Why was I in a dining hall with all of these crazy people? Why couldn't I be with normal people?

I felt guilty thinking that way. A few months ago, I'd been like these "crazy" people. I would be one of them today but for the grace of God.

Finally, someone came and wheeled me back to my room.

I asked the aide, "Is anyone going to get that poor lady who recites nursery rhymes?"

"As soon as possible," she said. "We're so busy at this time of the morning. Everyone needs to go back at the same time and then be helped to the toilet."

"I just want to take a nap."

When we got back to my room, the aide helped me get into bed and pulled the covers around me.

I sighed and fell into a delicious sleep.

♦ ♦ ♦

After lunch I sat in my wheelchair, reading a book.

"Susie?"

In the doorway stood my childhood friend, Barb, whom I hadn't seen since my birthday a couple of weeks before in the hospital. And beside Barb was Nancy, another friend I'd grown up with.

"It's so great to see you both. Nancy, aren't you here from Arizona?"

The three of us had just started catching up when a glum-looking young man stepped into my room.

"You want to go down to the physical therapy room?" he asked, sounding doubtful.

"No, my friends just got here, and I want to talk to them."

"Okay." He slumped out of the room, and Barb and Nancy wheeled me outside into the bright sunshine.

Later, after I finished dinner and waited twenty minutes for someone to wheel me back to my room. I felt a bit irritated about the wait, and I was getting ready to ask that my helper put me in bed right away when she walked up to my dresser. "Oh," she said. With wide eyes, she picked up the picture of my guru, walking in the gardens of her ashram in India. The aide got a gentle smile on her face.

"Who is this?" she asked.

"That's my guru." I felt my shoulders relax, and I let out a long breath.

"So much love coming from her."

"I feel it too," I said, looking at this aide with a new affinity. She was attractive with thick black hair and light brown skin. "What's your name?" I asked.

"Rosa."

We kept on talking as she efficiently helped me onto the toilet seat.

"Okay," she said. "Be right back."

"No, Rosa, don't leave me," I called out, but she hurried away.

I put my forehead into my hands and laughed.

We had been talking about such an uplifting subject, but now I was stuck on a hard toilet seat. It is so hard to depend on someone else for every move you make! And I waited on that toilet for nearly half an hour, with my bottom hurting more as each moment ticked away.

I realized that I'd better stop turning down physical therapy if I ever wanted to be strong enough to move through my life on my own steam—like getting off of this damn toilet!

♦   ♦   ♦

The next morning a new physical therapist came to my room, and seeing her, I smiled. "I'm ready for you," I said.

She rolled me down the hall past some colorful drawings that were displayed on the walls. "Is that some art by the patients here?" I asked.

"It sure is. We offer an art class here as a part of our occupational therapy program."

"And what is that big gray machine by the wall that I keep passing?"

"That's an ice machine."

"Do the aides come and get ice out every morning about four-thirty?"

"Probably. So that everyone can have nice cold water to drink."

"I was wondering what that loud smashing sound was. But the water is good. And as long as we're on the subject of strange noises, why are there so many horns honking outside of my window? Is traffic really that bad?"

She paused for a moment and then said, "The Seattle teachers are on strike and picketing out front. You're most likely hearing drivers honking to support them."

Things in this new world were beginning to make sense.

I was brought into a small room with bright paint and shiny laminate flooring. Therapists were sitting at school-sized desks working on their computers and one patient was lying on the floor getting what looked like range of motion therapy. I was helped onto a bicycle exercise machine. My physical therapist set some dials and had me start pedaling.

"Whoa, this is hard. It feels like I'm going uphill, and my legs are really weak, you know. I was in bed for over five weeks."

As she adjusted my machine, and it felt a little easier.

"You had viral encephalitis, didn't you?"

I thought for a moment. "Yeah, I think that's what I had."

"No wonder your legs are weak."

My shoulders tensed and my stomach clenched with an icy fear.

What did she mean by that? Was something wrong with my brain? Wasn't I going to walk again? Would I always need a walker? How was I going to get up and down the stairs in my house?

Anxiety gripped me as I contemplated a bleak and lonely future trapped in my house.

Chapter 19

PROTECTION

It was my second week in rehab and the third week of September. The trees were beginning to turn crimson and gold. The sky had gone from a hazy cerulean to the sharp blue sky of a northwest autumn. I was sitting in my room, reading a book after my physical therapy workout when a dear friend appeared in my doorway.

"Katherine," I said, "it's so good to see you! Pull up a chair. I don't remember a lot about being in the hospital, but you didn't visit, right?

"No, I wasn't able to visit you when you were in the hospital because I was at the ashram in New York. I had finally gotten a chance to fly there and work on a project that lasted an entire month."

"Well, that must have been wonderful."

"It's what I've been waiting for ever since I moved back to Seattle," she said in a soft voice.

Katherine had lived and worked full time in the New York meditation ashram for fourteen years before she'd moved back home to Seattle. I never knew exactly why she'd returned—perhaps to be closer to her two adult sons.

"I can stay here only a little while, but I've got something for you." Katherine handed me a small silk bag closed with a drawstring. I pulled out a lovely bracelet with light orange oval-shaped beads.

"This is gorgeous."

"It's a *rakhi* bracelet."

"Oh yeah, that's right, Rakhi Day was in August."

Rakhi Day, or *Raksha Bandhan,* is celebrated every year in India. Traditionally, on this day a sister ties a bracelet made from woven threads on her brother's wrist. The *rakhi* is a gift to him, and he, in turn, promises to give his sister his protection throughout life. On our spiritual path we give and receive *rakhi* bracelets with anyone who is special to us.

"Thank you, Katherine. What a sweet gift."

"It's not from me," she said. "It's from the guru."

"What? I can't believe it! How did that happen?"

"Let me tell you this little story," Katherine said, leaning forward in her chair. "It was the evening of Rakhi Day, and I was going back to my room after dinner. Someone called me over and said the guru was giving rakhi bracelets and I should go and get mine. She was sitting on the roof watching the moon rise. Susan, I was just thrilled. It was a lovely warm evening, and the guru looked so beautiful sitting in her chair in her shimmering orange robes. There was a table with *rakhi* bracelets on them, and we were invited to pick one. After we chose, the guru asked all of us if we knew anyone who might like a bracelet. I raised my hand and answered, 'Yes, I do. My friend Susan Bruzas has been quite ill, and I know she'd really appreciate one.' Then the guru told me to come and choose one for you."

"Oh, Katherine."

Katherine looked at me intently. "You know when the guru gives us a *rakhi*, it is both a promise of protection and a vow from us to protect our beautiful path."

I sighed, imagining what it must have been like to sit on the roof with our guru, the full moon rising, pale yellow in the sky, gradually turning silver and illuminating all the faces turned toward its cool soothing presence. It was perfect to receive a gift symbolizing protection from the guru.

And it was true that I'd felt safe throughout my illness, despite the initial dire diagnosis that I had metastasized brain cancer.

"Katherine, this means so much to me. Thank you for thinking of me." I put the bracelet on and felt its smooth beads. A stillness vibrated within me and seemed to fill the room.

Katherine looked at me with compassion and said, "Do you want me to tell the organizer for the India trip that you won't be going?"

"What?" I said, catching my breath at the sudden switch in mood. "Right, India. But I could still get better before the trip!"

"There's just not enough time," she said.

I started to protest, but then I stopped. She was probably right. Even if I managed to make it to India, what if I got sick again while I was there? I didn't want to end up needing to be rescued from half-way around the world.

"You're probably right," I said. "Okay, go ahead and tell them."

After Katherine left, I fingered the beads on my wrist.

◆　◆　◆

I was disappointed that I wouldn't be going on the trip to India. I'd put a lot of prep work into it, and I would have been traveling with a wonderful group of people.

Still, I felt a sense of wonder at what I'd just been through. I had been so protected. A tidal wave of misfortune had moved inexorably toward me, and I had kept my head up as it roared over me. I was not completely unscathed perhaps, but I was essentially unharmed.

It occurred to me that, if the timing had been just two days later, I would have been stricken with encephalitis as I was driving to Montana to see Lily. What would have happened then?

I shivered, remembering the sharp turns going over the three mountain passes on the way to Missoula. I closed my eyes and silently thanked God.

At dinner that night, I was once again placed with a patient who wouldn't, or couldn't, communicate. He was a handsome man with lots of silvery hair. I had sat with him a couple of times before. We hadn't talked to each other before, but I thought why not give it a try?

"Hi," I said. "How are you this evening?"

He stared at me with his piercing blue eyes and didn't say a word.

Oh no, here we go again.

"Looks like a good dessert," I said, pointing to the chocolate cake.

He continued looking at me, unblinking and silent.

I sighed and looked toward the cheerful talkative group of women I had seen sitting together at every meal since I'd arrived.

As usual, there was no room for me.

I felt a heaviness in my chest. After everything I'd been through, I still felt envy for these chattering, chirping women who were sitting together. I couldn't believe that I still felt left out.

It was a familiar emotion. I'd felt isolated for many years. The feeling had faded with the full-time job of being a single parent of two little girls. After the kids had grown up and moved away, loneliness had seeped back into my life. Many days I'd sat in my recliner staring out my living room window, watching my neighbors working in their yards and playing with their children. I'd think about the time I had worked as a speech therapist in nursing homes where the patients sat alone, staring out the window. Those patients would tell me that their children lived far away and were busy with their own lives.

Would I end up that way myself?

I took a deep breath into this dense sadness, willing it to dissolve. I gave myself a little pep talk: "For God's sake, Susan! You've had so many visitors and well-wishers. So what if you're sitting with people who can't talk. Come on, at least *you* can talk!"

I looked at the handsome man who was sitting across from me at our table—still staring at me, still saying nothing.

"Bye," I said to him in a cheerful voice. "Have a good evening."

I turned away and, for the first time, wheeled myself all the way back to my room and up to my bed. I pushed the button to raise the mattress to the right height, and then I scooted from the wheelchair onto the bed.

Feeling proud, though a bit tired and chilled, I pulled a blanket around me. My body felt heavy. I dropped off to sleep for a moment, but then I awoke with a start, feeling kind of sick. What was going on? I figured that I might need some help after all.

I pressed the call button and waited. I could hear the chime of another person's request, and the murmur of patients going back to their rooms. I felt my forehead with the inside of my wrist. It felt hot. I fell into an uneasy sleep.

I had a funny dream in which I couldn't figure out some math problem. The numbers just wouldn't add up, and I thought I was going to get in trouble. I was going to flunk. It seemed I had to figure this out.

The next thing I heard was, "Susan? Are you okay? Come on, honey, wake up."

When I opened my eyes, Rosa was looking at me intently.

"Oh Rosa, I was having a nightmare. I'm so glad you're here. I feel sick. Sort of cold, and then hot and shaky."

She took my temperature. "You have a fever of 103. I'll be right back."

In a few minutes the on-call doctor came in with assistants following. They wheeled in a miniature x-ray machine. The doctor listened with his stethoscope to my lungs and took my temperature again.

"It's high," he said, his eyes narrowed with worry. "How are you feeling?"

"Like I have the flu, I guess. Am I all right? Will I have to go back to the hospital?"

"Let's take a picture of your lungs right now and then do some blood tests."

Everybody moved fast after that, leaving me feeling scared that this was a real emergency. The nurse gave me a shot full of antibiotics.

I asked again if I would have to go back to Virginia Mason.

No one would answer.

Chapter 20

LEARNING THE SKILLS OF LIVING

L ater that night, the room light came on, waking me from a peaceful sleep.

"Your temperature is coming down," the attendant said. "Are you feeling better?"

I told her, "I don't know if it's the placebo effect. . . Or is it the halo effect? No, the halo effect is when a doctor is nice to a patient, and then the patient does better medically. I don't think it's that!" Then I was worried that she might think I didn't think she was nice, so I added, "Not that the kindness of the medical people hasn't had a positive effect on me. It has."

At this, the aide's eyebrows came together as if she was finding my rambling worrisome. Maybe she saw it as an indication that I wasn't out of the woods yet. I thought I'd better get back on topic.

"Anyway," I said, "I don't know if it's the placebo effect, but right after I got the shot of antibiotics, I felt a lot better." I paused. "I know I'm going on and on," I said. "It's just that I am really relieved. I was afraid I'd have to go back to the hospital."

"Not if your temp stays down," she said. She smiled reassuringly.

"I sure hope it does."

"No worries. We'll be checking on you during the night."

With the lights back off, I listened to the sweet melody of my mantra being sung by my beloved guru. Drifting off to sleep, I remembered my mom's soothing touch on my forehead when I had been ill as a child. Mom would always reassure me that I was getting better. She'd say, "No more fever, honey. You're cool as a cucumber."

The next time I was awakened that night, my hand was being lifted gently to slip on a pulse oximeter. I held the back of my hand to my head. "Cool as a cucumber," I said.

♦　♦　♦

The next morning, I awoke to another bright autumn day. I pushed my covers back and stretched out my arms toward the ceiling. My strength was coming back, and I wanted to go home.

After breakfast, the physical therapist held lightly to the gait belt as I shuffled up and down the halls with the walker. Gathering my courage I said, "I want to learn to go upstairs with my walker."

She looked at me for a moment. "Okay, that's great," she said. "Hoping to go home soon?"

"Yeah, I am. And to even get into my house I have to go up some stairs. I live in a split-level house. There are two small flights leading up to the front door, and then, once you're inside, a long flight to the living room. When I had hip replacement surgery, I was able to use crutches. But I can't do that now. So, I need to start practicing on a walker."

"Okay, let's find some stairs, and I'll teach you."

We approached the bottom of a long flight of stairs. Apprehension fluttered through my stomach like frightened birds.

But I was going to do this. I straightened my shoulders and took a deep breath. I said, "Okay, let's go for it."

"Do your stairs have a railing?"

"Uh, let's see. I think so." Did they? "Wait a minute," I told her. I closed my eyes for a moment and tried to visualize what the front of my house looked like. It had been so long, and how carefully had I ever looked at it?

I said, "Okay, the first three front steps do not have a railing. Then there's a little. . .um, what do you call it?" I felt myself growing warm with embarrassment. Why couldn't I find the words to describe this simple. . .*thing*?

"A landing?"

"Well, maybe. There's a little concrete slab that has room for planters, and you have to turn and walk up about five more steps to the door. The last five steps have a railing. Then you go in the front door and there's a long flight of stairs into the living room, and these, too, have a railing."

"Okay, got it. Since some of the stairs don't have railings, we'll practice going up with both hands on the walker. First let's walk up closer to the stairs. Now skip the first step and put the first two legs of your walker, up to the second step."

I lifted the walker and followed her instructions feeling her grip on the gait belt against my back. It was comforting to know she could stabilize me if I started to lose my balance.

"Now, with your weight on the front of your walker, put your right foot on the first step. Then the next foot."

For a moment I froze. My hands turned pale as I gripped the front bar. I stared at the step that was in front of me and then took a deep breath. Inwardly I repeated my mantra.

I made it up the first step.

Now, there was a second step. I told myself not to look up. I told myself to breathe. In this way, I made it up the ten steps to the landing.

"I did it," I said, sighing with relief.

"Yes, nice job," the PT told me. "Ready for the next steps?"

I looked up. Oh my God, there were at least ten more stairs.

♦　♦　♦

"I think you can do it," the PT said, smiling.

I bit my lip. The truth was that I could barely make it up a whole flight of stairs even when I was completely healthy!

"Okay," I said, but my voice was quaking.

"It is okay," she said. "I'll be right here."

I took a deep breath.

"Feeling alright?" the PT asked me. "You're not dizzy or anything?"

"Just a bit tired."

But little by little, with the walker clunking up each step, I finally reached the second-floor landing.

"You made it," the PT said.

"I feel like I just climbed a mountain!"

There was no prize at the top, however, and after just a few minutes, it was time to go back down again. Once again, I was telling myself that I could do this. For the descent, the PT showed me how to close the walker and turn it sideways; how to hold the walker with my left hand and the railing with my right hand.

It was complicated, but I managed to follow her instructions, and take my first step down. My shoulders tensed and I forgot to breathe as I leaned my body forward toward the next stair down— but the PT was standing in front of me, and she had her hands on my shoulders for support.

After a brief eternity and a lot of work, I got to the bottom.

"Oh, my God," I said. "I can't believe we did it."

"I had no doubt we would," my helper said.

The question was, how would I ever be able to get up and down my front stairs at home—by myself!

Back at my room, I found a note on my door saying a social worker wanted to meet with me to talk about my going home. So, that might be happening soon. I got on the phone and set up an appointment for later in the day.

Then I sat on my bed and stared out the window, feeling a little overwhelmed. On the tree outside, the leaves were turning the color of burgundy. It was the end of September. I hadn't been home for seven weeks. I had lived on my own for years. Now, I had no idea how I was going to take care of myself. How would I shop for groceries? Do my laundry? Take care of my cat? The very thought made my stomach roil, and I bit my lip until it hurt.

Then I tried some positive self-talk: Come on, Susan. Breathe. Talk to the social worker about all of this. That's what the meeting is about.

My phone chimed with a notification that I was scheduled for a shower soon—my first since I'd been at rehab. Even though I had given myself a shower in the hospital, that wasn't allowed here. It had taken several steps to schedule this upcoming shower: I'd had to find a room with a shower and sign up for one of the few time slots that were available.

I felt fortunate to have a new pair of sweatpants and bright purple T-shirt Val had given to me as a belated birthday present. Not only would I be getting clean, but I'd be putting on new clothes.

An attendant came to give me my shower.

"Hello, Susan," she said, "I'm Jean. Ready for the shower?"

"Oh, you bet I am. I can't wait."

We walked down the hall chatting away as if we were two birds chirping back and forth. The shower took place in a large room that was cluttered with buckets and stacks of towels. I stripped out of my clothes, clutched the grab bars, and lowered myself down onto a raised toilet seat directly underneath a shower head, which was sticking out of the wall.

The attendant talked in a cheerful voice as her gentle hands washed my hair and body with soap that smelled like Ivory. I felt myself completely relax with the feeling of warm, soothing water flowing over me. I was grateful a friend had sent a hairdresser to cut and neaten my long shaggy hair.

Back in my room, I dried and curled my hair and dressed in my new clothes. I looked forward showing off my new look at dinner.

This it would be the first meal for which I would be out of a wheelchair and using a walker.

As I entered the dining hall, I shuffled my walker over to the round table full of the women who were so friendly and talkative. A few of the regular group had been able to go home leaving a space for me to join them. I stood smiling down at them feeling six feet tall.

"Well, don't you look great," Judy said. She had MS and had been at rehab for several weeks after taking a fall.

The rest of the women murmured their compliments.

"Why thank you," I said.

"Going home soon?" Delores asked. She was wearing a flowery dress and was about to go home herself.

"I have a meeting with the social worker soon, and we're going to discuss it. I practiced going up and down stairs today."

I pulled out the plastic chair to sit down. Usually, I had used a wheelchair. The dining table chair looked a long way down. There were no arms on the chair to help me balance.

Seeing my bewilderment, one of the women called to an attendant to find a chair with arms so that I could manage this maneuver.

Once someone had pulled up a chair for me, I aimed myself toward it and dropped heavily into the seat.

A few of the women watching me gasped. "You almost fell and hurt yourself," one of them told me. "You ought to be more careful. Do you want to spend a few more weeks here?"

I cringed inside with a mixture of shame and embarrassment. As the conversation resumed, I sat in silence chastising myself.

I had no idea how I was going to get out of this chair and up to my walker! Why hadn't I just come in with my wheelchair? And after I went home, how was I going to sit down and get up there? Was my furniture high enough off the ground? What height was my bed? What if I fell when I was alone at home?

With questions swirling in my mind, I ate my food, tasting noth-ing.

Chapter 21

IS THIS A TEST?

Why didn't this social worker get off the phone?

I had a 9:00 a.m. appointment with the social worker to discuss if, and when, I'd be going home. It was our second meeting. The first time we got together, we'd talked about my fears. I was worried about being alone in my house. I was also worried about getting up and downstairs to answer the front door. I was worried about doing laundry and getting groceries. She'd promised to look into the possibility of my staying on for a couple of weeks in one of rehab's independent cottages.

The more I thought about it, the more I wanted to stay in one of those pretty little cottages. They were white, and they had big window boxes full of red geraniums. I loved the flowers. The cottage residents get to eat in the dining hall, and they were always talking and laughing when they took their meals.

It was 9:08, and the social worker was still on the phone.

She was the one who had set the time for this appointment. First, she was five minutes late and then, once she'd arrived, she'd answered the phone. Why had she answered it? She could see me sitting here. Now, I looked at her intently and thought, *Hang up!* Perhaps I should just pace back and forth. That would be quite dramatic with a walker.

I took a deep breath and told myself, *Lighten up!*

Once I'd had that thought, the social worker looked up, gave me a smile, and waved.

I took another breath and waved back.

A few minutes later, I was sitting across from her and asking her, "Can I stay?"

"Well, I looked into you moving to the cottages for a while," she said, shuffling some papers.

"Uh-huh."

"You have really good insurance. But it's not going to work out."

"Really? Why?" I asked, trying to swallow my disappointment.

"The average age is eighty-two. You're . . . how old?"

"Um, sixty-seven—no, sixty-eight."

"Yes, that's right." She looked at me, her blue eyes reflecting concern. "Do you have anyone who could stay with you for a while?"

"My youngest daughter is coming for a kind of vacation with my six-year-old grandson and staying at my house for a week sometime in the last week of September. I forget the exact date."

"Do you have any other family?"

"My older daughter, Lily, has told me she would come for a little longer depending on how much time she can get off work."

"That would be good," she said, sipping some coffee out of a blue chipped mug.

"But I still have a little bit of trouble getting off the chairs in the dining hall," I went on. "And my living room couch is pretty low—and I don't even know how high my bed is." My voice was getting higher pitched and more intense the longer I spoke.

"Give me a moment and I can look up some sites for you to get adaptive equipment."

While I waited for her to finish her research, I looked out the office window and watched a handsome dark-haired man walk by, holding the arm of a resident named Rose.

It was Ronnie—who was so sweet to Rose, his mom.

Ronnie liked sitting with the ladies in the dining hall and regaling us with stories about Rose, who seemed to have a special dispensation to live in our rehab section. Every day as I went by her room, I would see her sitting by a round mirror putting on pretty earrings and powdering her nose. Her face always lit up when she saw her son.

I ached to see my own kids. Alena told me she'd visited for a week when I was in the hospital, but I had no memory of it.

"Here are some websites for shower stools, raised toilets, and even chairs that lift you, like the one you have here in your room," she said, writing the links down on a sticky note.

"I guess I could get it all together and arrange for my family to stay for a while. Maybe my sister could come too."

"Okay," the social worker said. "Let's say at the end of this week, we'll arrange transportation to take you home."

That was Friday. Okay, I had some research to do, some phone calls to make.

◆ ◆ ◆

I called Lily the next morning. She was coming, and for two weeks. I was thrilled!

"I think I can get the time off work," she said, "but I'll still need to make my rent. Do you think you can help with that, since I'll be missing both my hourly pay and my tips?"

"Oh, sure," I told her. I had all the money I'd saved for my trip to India. I wouldn't be going on that—so, yes, I could help my daughter.

"I have some really good recipes I can try on you," Lily said. She giggled. "Gotta get you fattened up," she said.

"Hah! Not really, but it will be great to have some home-cooked meals. I'm getting a little tired of this bland institutional food."

"Do you have someone staying with you before I come?"

"Alena is coming," I said. "But my first night at home, I'll be by myself."

"Mom, that's not good. You're still on a walker. What if you fall?"

"I know," I told her. "It will be kind of scary after being with people for so long. But Val and Jenny will be there for the day, and I'll only be by myself for the night. Alena and Rowan will be coming from the airport the next morning."

After a few more minutes of my reassuring Lily that I'd be all right, we said goodbye. I could hardly wait to see both of my girls. I could hardly wait to get out of rehab. It was just a couple of days away. What would it be like to actually be by myself? It seemed like eons of time had passed since I'd headed out to the meditation center to celebrate Gurupurnima.

I had been doing all I could to prepare for going home. I'd tried calling around to find a power lift recliner, but they were way too expensive. I decided that I would put wide pillows on my couch and then push myself to standing.

I'd also made a frantic call to my neighbor, Diane, asking her to measure the distance between the floor and the top of the mattress on my bed. I had to be sure I could boost myself from the bed to my walker. She'd run right over to my house and checked. Thank God, my bed was high enough. And thank God for Diane.

◆ ◆ ◆

My last day in rehab dawned cool and cloudy. It was typical for Seattle to have the blue skies and hot temperatures of summer disappear overnight. I hadn't realized that it was already September 26, two days after the official beginning of fall.

I had my final meal with my rehab friends. One member of our group had gone home recently, her infected leg wound totally healed. I remembered her standing straight without her walker. She had put on a loose flowery dress and bright red lipstick to celebrate. "You look fabulous," I'd told her. A smile lit her face in reply. She proudly walked away, turning at the door to wave at us.

Now, it was my turn. With a combination of wistfulness and sincerity, I was congratulated.

"Where do you live?" Judy asked.

"In a house close to Lake City. It's a split level, but I think I can get up the stairs."

"Big?"

"Sort of. My daughters are coming to help out, though. Where do you live?"

"I have a condo close to University Village." That was also an upscale neighborhood.

There was brief silence. I knew that some of the women sitting at the table couldn't work and that they lived in apartments funded by city agencies. There was a moment of silence.

We were joined by a nice-looking man with silver hair and bright blue eyes. It was the strange guy I'd sat with a few times at the hospital—the one who never said a word.

"Where are you from?" someone asked him.

"Portland," he said, glancing at me.

So, he could actually talk!

"Are you still working?" Judy queried.

"I'm a retired dentist. I do teach some classes at Portland State University."

"I took a summer class there," I said. "It was in phonetics, a credit I needed for my BA in speech therapy. The class was hard, but I had a good teacher. and I liked taking the bus to downtown Portland."

Everyone was still talking when I said goodbye. About a half an hour later, Judy came to my room.

"All packed?" she asked.

"Yes. A friend came by and helped. Another friend took all my stuff to my house."

"I just wanted to tell you what the dentist said after you left."

"Oh? What?"

"He's really shy and has been trying to get up his nerve to get your phone number so he could give you a call and set up a date or something. When you left, he said, 'We're finally talking, and she's leaving. I missed my chance.'"

"You're kidding me! Whenever I sat at his table, he'd just stare at me. I thought he couldn't talk and was surprised when I saw you two having a conversation."

"No, he was in rehab to recover from knee surgery. There's nothing wrong with his brain."

I thanked her for letting me know. After Judy said goodbye again, I sat staring out the window. I was really surprised to hear all of this about the silver-haired man. I suppose that I could have tried harder to engage him in a conversation. But I'd thought it was creepy that he just stared at me and didn't say anything.

For a moment I considered the possibility of trying to find him or to get his name. But then I realized that I wasn't interested in dating anyone. It had been too long.

◆ ◆ ◆

In the early afternoon, my cabulance arrived. The sun broke through just as I was wheeled through the facility's front door.

I was going home. I could barely fathom it!

Once I was settled in the vehicle, we started off. We turned left out of the parking lot, and I gazed at the scenery, utterly fascinated. I hadn't been anywhere or seen anything other than the views from my hospital and rehab rooms for eight weeks.

It felt surreal, like I was watching a movie. Where was I, anyway?

I peered out of the driver's window. We turned right on a busy street which said 135.

"One thirty-fifth!" I said. "I can't believe that all this time, I've been only a few miles from my own home. We're going to turn left on Fifteenth Northeast, and then we'll almost be there."

"Yep," the driver said. "We're really close."

As my heart filled with happiness, I watched as we turned and headed down the hill.

Now, we were going over I-5. All of the traffic was backed up. I hadn't missed that! But I couldn't wait until I could drive again. And there was the old Safeway. Oh my gosh, we were turning onto my street. I wondered if my neighbor Janet and her girls were home.

We pulled into the driveway, and I looked up at my 1960s home with its white wooden siding and brown trim. The grass was still brown from the hot summer, but the yellow climbing roses were flourishing. I smiled as the driver wheeled me out the back doors and down a ramp. Mary Lou was waiting in the driveway with a frown on her face.

"Mary Lou!" I exclaimed. "I didn't know you were going to be here!"

I don't know why, but I felt a little irritated. Mary Lou had thought I should hire a mutual friend to stay with me for this first night home—and I hadn't felt that I should need to pay a friend to stay with me.

"I wasn't going to let you get home by yourself."

The driver handed me my walker, and I pushed it to the bottom of the three flights of stairs. I needed to climb those stairs to get to the living area of my house. Mary Lou and the driver stood watching me, not saying a word. No words of encouragement. No sign of physical support.

For God's sake. Was this a test?

Determined, I clunked one side of the walker onto the first step. . .

Chapter 22

CHOCOLATE CHIP COOKIES, A VEGGIE BURGER, AND FRIENDS

Clunk-slap-clunk sounded the walker as I made my way through the front door and up the long flight of stairs into my living room.

I whispered my mantra at each step, giving myself small boosts of confidence. As I approached the last step, I had a sudden image of almost falling. It appeared in my mind like a slow-motion movie. Five years before, I had just returned from a surgery on my foot, and I was using crutches to navigate the steps. I had just boosted myself up to the landing when I began to feel myself tipping backward.

"L-e-e-ena," my voice had quivered my daughter's nickname while my body wobbled back and forth.

"You're okay, Mom," she said. "You're okay." And I was—because in the last second, I'd regained my balance and my confidence.

Once again, the fateful last step was before me. This time the walker, which was just as clumsy as it felt, gave me more stability than the crutches had. I made the final step with no problem at all.

"I'm here," I said with a sigh of relief.

Mary Lou and the driver then carried bags and boxes up the stairs, and I sat down on top of the cushions that were piled on the couch. I looked around. My domain seemed neglected. The air was stale, and it held the faint smell of dry cat food—as if the windows hadn't been opened for a while. I realized that once my family had returned to their homes—about a month ago—no one but my neighbor had been in the house, and she'd come only to feed the cat.

William. Where was he anyway? I hadn't seen him for two months.

"William," I called. "William!"

The cat did not appear. Perhaps he was sound asleep on my bed. Then I heard him purring.

I looked around, and there he was peering at me, his gray and white head raised from the seat of the leather chair. He was lying on top of a plaid wool blanket, which was just covered with cat hair.

"There you are. Come on, kitty. Come over here and see me."

I called to William several times, but he didn't budge.

"I know you think I deserted you. That's okay. I'll come over and pet you in a little while."

Mary Lou sat down with a sigh after taking my suitcase to my bedroom. I looked at her tired face and the irritation I'd been harboring toward her evaporated.

She had done so much for me! How could I feel anything but gratitude?

"Are you hungry, Susan? Is there anything in the fridge?"

"Just some cream for my tea."

"What do you feel like eating? I could run and pick you up something."

"Wow, that's really nice of you. Actually, I've been imagining eating a Kidd Valley Garden Burger and french fries with tartar sauce."

"Okay. I could run up to the one on Aurora and get one." She looked around the living area. "Will you be all right here on your own? Can you get to the bathroom and the bedroom?"

"Val and her husband are bringing over a few groceries and a raised toilet seat. They should be here pretty soon. And why don't I experiment with getting up from the couch. After getting up those stairs, this should be nothing!"

I didn't feel as confident as I sounded. It was another test during which Mary Lou would be staring at me, assessing me.

I told myself to chill. I had just been reminding myself what a good friend Mary Lou had always been.

So, I took a breath and focused on the walker in front of me. I put my hands next to my body and used them to push. Instead of propelling my body up, my hands sank down, going deeper into the couch. I fell back down, and frustration tinged with embarrassment burned in my stomach.

But I could do better than this. What was it I had practiced earlier? There were steps. I closed my eyes and concentrated on remembering the steps.

"Let's see," I said. "Move to the end of the chair, put one foot a little forward, the opposite hand on the walker, and then push."

"That sounds good," Mary Lou said.

"Okay. One. . . two. . . three."

This time I made it. I gave Mary Lou a triumphant smile.

"You did it, Susan. Great! Let's take a look at your bed."

The bed was just the right height and very simple to get on. I stretched out for a moment on the mattress.

"It's going to be wonderful to sleep here again. I won't get woken up at 4:30 in the morning by the sound of the assistants down the hall stabbing the ice blocks to make chips. And when I wake up, I'll be able to hear the birds chirping and stare at my sweet gum tree out of the window."

"I bet it will be a relief," Mary Lou said. "Are you sure you'll be all right by yourself tonight?"

"It will be a little weird, but I'll be good."

She patted my knee and said, "Let's see you get up, and then I'll go get that veggie burger."

I had no problem at all getting off my bed and into the living room, so Mary Lou headed out to get dinner.

♦ ♦ ♦

A few minutes later there was a knock at the front door. OMG! Was I going to have to schlep downstairs to answer it?

Then I heard, "Hello? Susie Q?"

It was Val. "Wow," I said. "I didn't expect you so soon."

"We wanted to bring your stuff."

Val and her husband trooped upstairs, carrying bags and a big white toilet seat.

Mike tore open the packaging for the toilet, and I gave him a sheepish smile. "Are you ready for this adventure?" I asked him.

"I even brought my tools," he said, heading for the bathroom.

"Hello-o-o-o-o-o!"

"Up here, Jenster," Val responded.

My friend Jenny handed me a plate of chocolate chip cookies—my favorite! "Thank you, Jenny," I told her. "This is really nice of you!"

We all sat there, munching cookies and chatting about nothing much at all. It felt almost normal, like I hadn't been sick for eight weeks.

Before I knew it, Mary Lou was handing me my garden burger, I'd eaten it, and everyone was saying their goodbyes. Mary Lou promised to pick up my daughter and grandson at the airport the next day. They would be here for a week.

It was going to be so good to have them all to myself.

I waved to Mary Lou as she backed out of my driveway. The setting sun had turned the neighborhood houses shades of peach and coral. I sat down and looked around. The living room had an eerie silence. Long shadows were creeping over the landscape. I watched the sky grow darker and a feeling of apprehension made an unexpected appearance. The back of my neck prickled, and even though

I took a deep breath, it felt like there wasn't enough oxygen in the air.

"It's so stuffy in here," I said aloud, as my chest tightened. It felt as if there wasn't enough oxygen in the room—though I knew that there probably was. The thing is, I wanted to open a window, and I didn't have enough energy to get up and do that. But why was the nightfall bothering me so much?

I asked myself when it was that I'd begun dreading the end of the day. Scrolling back through the years, I realized that it started right after I'd graduated from college in the late sixties. My new husband had gone to officer's training school in Michigan, leaving me alone for the first time in my life. At that point, I grew so anxious about the ending of each day that I'd begged friends to let me stay the night with them. I'd be invited over for a friendly dinner and end up sleeping on the couch. As time went on, I grew accustomed to living alone, and I stopped embarrassing myself by being needy with my friends.

Was that what was happening now? Was I feeling alone again? Maybe. I'd felt safe in the hospital and rehab because there was always someone to ring if I was scared. What was going to happen now that I was here on my own?

Gradually I began to feel better. I could see Diane across the street, scurrying around in her living room. She was such a busy bee. And I knew behind the windows of other homes were neighbors who would come to help if I called. I had all of their phone numbers.

I pushed my walker into my bedroom and pulled some musty-smelling pajamas from my dresser drawer. The raised toilet was easy to get on and off. Soon, I climbed into bed and pulled my quilt up. It felt good to be in my own bed.

"William," I called. "William, I'm home. Come here and jump on up."

No William. He was really mad at me.

I let out a long breath and turned off the light. As I drifted off to sleep, I realized that I'd forgotten to turn the mantra on my iPhone.

◆　◆　◆

Sometime later I woke up. It was really dark, which surprised me because I thought I'd put on a light in the hallway before I went to bed. There wasn't even any ambient light coming from the sky or streetlights across the street.

Then it occurred to me that no streetlights are visible from my bedroom. Where was I? I realized then that I was standing up. Okay, but where?

I looked around and saw the outlines of my two couches, coffee table, and reclining chair.

Oh my God, I was in the living room! Had I been walking in my sleep? I hadn't walked in my sleep since I was fifteen. It didn't even occur to me that I didn't have my walker.

Putting my hands out, I felt my way to the hall. Finding the switch on the wall, I turned on the light. Nothing happened. I tried again, flicking the switch off and on. No light. This seemed familiar somehow.

Had the power gone off? There hadn't been any high winds to knock out power lines. Had someone cut them?

Then it occurred to me that this had happened before. I might be having one of my recurring lucid dreams. Or it might be that my spirit was actually floating around while my body was still sleeping.

Oh, my God! What if my soul couldn't get back to my body? I might be stuck in this dark place forever.

I figured that whether this was a lucid dream or astral travel, what I had to do was to get back to my bedroom. If I could just get back to my sleeping body, I could wake myself up. I figured that I'd better go back to the bedroom right now, or else I might not wake up at all!

Chapter 23

WIGGLING BLACK WORMS

I looked down but saw only darkness. Where were my feet? I sensed that I had hands and tried waving them around in the inky black, but still I could see nothing. My blood felt icy cold. I was frightened. Why couldn't I see?

Somehow, I found myself in my bedroom. Here was my bedside lamp—my mother's beautiful stained-glass lamp. Would I be able to turn it on? Praying that I could, I caught hold of the chain and pulled it down.

At that point, I opened my eyes. I was lying in my bed. My heart was beating hard in my chest, and I was rigid with fright. I could hear the distant sound of traffic and the rustling of the breeze in the tree outside my window. I felt like I had dropped here in the waking world from a place completely absent of light and sound. But was I awake? I held my breath, reached out, and pulled the chain of my bedside lamp. Now, the light came on.

I looked around the room, reassuring myself with the familiar details—the dresser, the pictures of my gurus on the wall, my clothes lying on the floor. I started taking deep breaths in and out, and this purposeful breathing slowed the pounding of my heart.

I looked for my phone. If I could just play the mantra on my phone, I knew the mantra would protect me from whatever it was that was happening.

So, with the light left on and the soothing sounds of the guru's voice singing the mantra, I sank into a peaceful sleep for the rest of the night.

♦ ♦ ♦

I was awakened by the cheerful, unrestrained song of a house finch. Birdsong had never penetrated the hospital or rehab facility. It had been so long since I'd heard the beautiful twittering of birds. I stretched my arms above my head and looked at the tree through my bedroom window. Dappled sunlight played on the star-shaped leaves that were beginning to turn a pale gold. Beyond the tree was a vibrant sapphire sky, reminding me of the singular beauty of the crisp fall days in the Pacific Northwest.

For a moment the darkness of that dream state from the night before settled over me. I shook it off, not wanting to spoil the excitement of waking up to a new day in my own home.

And weren't Alena and Rowan coming today? Yes! Now, that was something to get up for!

Excited, I pushed myself to the edge of the bed, grabbed the handle of the walker, and pulled myself up to standing.

♦ ♦ ♦

Before very long, Mary Lou pulled up in her little white Toyota with Alena and Rowan.

I couldn't remember the last time I'd seen Rowan. Was it last summer? Alena had been here this summer. She'd come to see me in the hospital—though I couldn't remember that at all.

When I heard Mary Lou use her key to open the front door, I called down from the living room level: "Hi, you guys! Alena and Rowan, welcome! I'm so happy you're here! Sorry, I can't come downstairs and greet you."

"Hi, Mom," Alena called out.

"Hi, Meemaw," Rowan said, bounding up the stairs with a big smile. My grandson had grown tall. His blue eyes were sparkling, and his hair was still blond from the summer.

I put my arm around him and gave him a side hug while holding onto my walker. "Wow, you're tall. You're in the first grade now? Second?"

"First, Meemaw. I'm six," he said, laughing.

"Mom, you're looking a lot better," Alena said, gazing at me intently.

I was puzzled.

She explained, "The last time we were together, you weren't doing so well."

I started sputtering: "What? Oh. Well. . . um, here. . .I mean, here I am."

Alena just smiled. "Yes, here we all are," she said. "I'm going to put our suitcases in the back bedroom."

Rowan had his own agenda: "I'm going to go visit the toy room," he said.

I hoped he wasn't expecting anything new. I hadn't done anything like that to prepare for him. "It's the same old toys I've had for a million years," I told him. "But your favorites are still there." Then I remembered my manners. "Mary Lou, please sit down," I said to my old friend. "Thanks so much for getting Alena and Rowan."

"It was just fine," Mary Lou said in a voice as mellifluous as a running stream. "The plane arrived on time, and everything went just fine." Then she looked at me closely. "So, how was your first night home after being away so long?"

I said that it was quiet and easy to be back at home—I didn't say a word about having the lucid dream or out-of-body experience or whatever it was that had come on me during the night. Why worry people!

In a few minutes, Alena joined us, and the three of us chatted while Rowan brought out box after box of toys and games.

◆　◆　◆

Soon, Mary Lou left, and Alena busied herself making the beds for herself and Rowan and fixing lunch for us all. Rowan and I were quite accustomed to playing together, and this time I made up a story about a yellow toy plane he'd found.

"The banana plane is sending down banana bombs," I called out. "Here it goes—five, four, three, two. . . bombs away! No, bananas away!"

Rowan laughed. He liked that. "I'll shoot it down," he yelled. "I'll make banana mush out of you. *Pew. Pew. Tat-tat-tat.*"

I was engaged in this play while sitting on top of a stack of pillows on the couch. It was more than I'd done in months, and I could feel my energy flagging.

After a while I told him, "I'm sorry, Rowan, but I'm bored." How could I have said that? "I mean I'm tired."

His body drooped with disappointment. For a few minutes, he sat in silence pushing a truck along the floor.

"Are you sad because Meemaw can't play, Rowan?" Alena asked with her eyes full of compassion.

He nodded, staring at the floor.

I didn't know what to say. "I'm really sorry, Rowan. I'm just tired." Then I told his mother, "I think I'm going to take a little nap."

"That's a good idea, Mom," Alena said. Then she turned to her son, "Rowan, how about we go to Third Place Bookstore? That would be fun for you."

"Okay," he said, cheering up a bit.

I understood that a little boy needs special care, but I was a little surprised that my daughter would leave me so soon after they'd arrived.

Alena may have picked up on that thought. She asked me, "You've got leftovers from lunch, don't you?"

"Um, yeah, I guess so."

"Okay then, we won't be gone long."

◆　◆　◆

They still weren't back when I got up from my nap. I got out the food I hadn't finished at lunch and ate a small supper, watching the light fade from the sky. I started remembering then the dream I'd had the night before of being lost in darkness. I had been thinking of it as a dream, but it was different from most dreams I'd had. There had been no light or sound and no dream characters. I couldn't decide whether I was sleepwalking or caught in a space that was separate from my body.

I hadn't walked in my sleep since I was fifteen. It occurred to me that maybe what had happened last night was an astral projection—my subtle body leaving my physical body.

At one point in my life, I used to have so much fun flying out of my body and going all over the place. I had read about this happening to other people—people whose subtle forms floated above their physical bodies while their doctors tried to revive them. I didn't know if this is what had happened to me. When I'd made my forays out into the night, I had never seen a vivid image of my physical body sleeping.

But whatever it was, I knew that last night had definitely not been fun.

Finally, I heard the car driving into the driveway and, soon after, the door to the garage opening. I talked for a few minutes with Alena and Rowan, but before long, I told them good night. It would have been nice to stay up longer, but I was exhausted.

◆　◆　◆

The next morning, I had an 8:00 a.m. appointment with two specialists. Alena went to get the car with Rowan right behind her. I was afraid to navigate the stairs to the front door with the walker. Instead, I scooted down each step on my rear end with one arm holding onto the railing. That brought me to the front door. On the steps outside, I didn't want to get my butt dirty, so I hung onto the railing while I carefully stepped down the concrete steps to the driveway. Then Alena handed me the walker, and I made my way to the car.

I noticed that Alena looked tired as she drove through the rush hour traffic to the medical buildings on Capitol Hill. I told her, "I'm sorry these appointments are so early. They were made for me when I was still in rehab."

"That's okay. We're just a little jet-lagged."

Looking at her, I wasn't sure if it was really jet lag. A veil of indifference or maybe resentment draped over her face. It occurred to me that Alena might not like being in the role of her mother's caretaker.

"Are you okay, Rowan?" she asked.

"Yeah, just hungry."

"I'll make sure I get you something at the snack bar."

Hearing this, I thought that I was probably being oversensitive. My daughter had to take care of her son first.

♦ ♦ ♦

Alena and Rowan stayed in the lobby playing cards as I made my way down a short hall to the neurologist's office. He was in his mid-forties, with curly brown hair and bright blue eyes, and when we first saw each other, he extended his hand toward me.

"Hi, I'm Dr. P.," he said.

"It's nice to meet you," I said, shaking his warm hand. "I'm Susan."

"Oh, we've met. You most likely don't remember." He looked at me with a wide smile on his face, like I wasn't quite real. "So, you're just out of rehab," he said. "How are you doing?"

"I'm doing great," I told him. "It's wonderful to be home and sleeping in my own bedroom. My daughter's staying with me for a while—and also my grandson. And then Lily, my older daughter, will be coming for two weeks. They're both great cooks. I'm going to get home physical therapy beginning this week. So, all in all, I'm doing very well."

As I spoke, his smile became radiant. "I can see from that explanation that your communication is fantastic," he said. "And you're getting around okay with a walker?"

"Yes." I had no intention of telling him about clinging to the rail that morning because I hadn't wanted to get my butt dirty.

Dr. P. checked my eyes and tested my reflexes, and then he looked at my chart. He told me that I had missed having a follow-up MRI at the hospital, so I could have one in the radiology clinic here.

I asked him what my last MRI had looked like.

"Would you like to see?" he said. "I have a copy of it right here."

"Sure. It might be interesting?"

He pulled it up on the computer, and then his eyebrows furrowed in a worried frown. "Are you sure you want to look at this?" he asked me. "It might be a little scary."

I told him it would be fine—and I would be fine—and then I sat in the chair next to his and looked at the image on the screen.

"This is the right side of your brain," he said. "These are bleeds, or hemorrhages, and the doctors could see that they were spreading."

What I was looking at resembled a whole lot of wiggling black worms. The doctor was telling me how they had ruled out lymphoma. I was having trouble listening to him. I couldn't stop staring at my brain with its writhing worms. Had the doctor just said "bleed"? Maybe it was "lesions." Or *hemorrhages?* I looked away from the computer and tried to breathe into the fear welling up inside me.

I couldn't imagine what had happened to me! What in hell had caused all of this?

The doctor was talking on: ". . .And then you woke up and were doing pretty well, considering. We figured it was the antiviral medicine working. And you're a fighter!"

"Oh, well. . ." I was stammering now, trying to focus on the doctor instead of that terrifying image. "Thank you. I guess I am a fighter. Uh, I have another appointment with the infectious disease specialist. I'm sorry, I have to get going."

"Oh," he said, looking a bit deflated. Then he said, "Of course. Let me walk you down the hall."

A few minutes later I was pushing my walker past a couple of doctors who were standing in their doorways.

"This is Susan Bruzas," Dr. P said, and the doctors looked at me as if I were a queen. I realized that they all seemed to know who I was. Had they seen me in the hospital? I gave them a little wave and said goodbye to my doctor.

◆　◆　◆

In the waiting room, I found Alena and Rowan playing Memory.

I told them, "I have another appointment with some doctor—I forgot his name—just across the hall." As I made my way across the long empty lobby, I had a flash of memory—a picture of black worms spreading in my brain. I took a shaky breath. What would the next doctor tell me? Just how sick had I been?

Chapter 24

A HAUNTED FEELING

"Hello, Susan. I'm Dr. Thottingal. I was one of your specialists."

The doctor's smile was genuine and his eyes warm. Whatever fear I was holding from seeing my MRI melted away. As he spoke, a vague memory of him drifted through my mind. He had been standing by the table in the beautiful hospital restaurant by the Sound. Nadine was sitting with me as we sipped coffee. "This is Dr. Thottingal. He's the infectious disease specialist who's consulting on your case," Dr. H had said.

But that didn't make any sense. What restaurant? And why would I think that this was the doctor who was introduced to me.

I let the memory go so I could concentrate on what *this* doctor— Dr. Paul Thottingal, who was standing right in front of me—was saying.

"You know, I consulted with many different doctors on your case trying to figure out what was going on with you. I sent them all of the test results and observations we had. Eventually, they got back to me and said, 'We don't know what's going on with her. Glad we're not in your shoes. Good luck!'"

We both laughed at that.

"But I think I that I read in the final hospital report that you said everyone should move away from the thinking that I had lymphoma and do some other testing," I said.

"True. And also keep you on the antiviral drug."

"And I woke up!"

"And you woke up," he said, smiling again. "And immediately afterward when we asked, you knew where you were, your name, when you were born!"

"I guess it's a miracle."

He looked at me intently. "It is."

Later, as we said goodbye, my heart filled with gratitude. What great doctors I'd had!

♦ ♦ ♦

"Mom, I have something to ask you." We had stopped for treats on the way back from my appointments and were sitting in line at the drive-through at Starbucks. It seemed like eons since I'd been there.

I looked at Alena and said, "Oh?"

"Remember when I told you I was dating someone new?"

"The last I remember you were going out with a few guys and had decided that you didn't want to date anyone for a while. You weren't ready, or something. Right?"

"Yes, but around the time you got sick, I decided to browse this online dating site, just for fun. And I started chatting back and forth with this really sweet, funny guy."

"Oh?"

"Yeah, and we finally had coffee and. . . Hold on." We had pulled up to the window. "Mom, what do you want?"

"A grande soy chai and a blueberry scone. It's been so long!"

A few minutes later, our order came.

"Here you go, Rowan," I said, handing him his brownie. Taking a sip of my chai, I savored the taste. "Oh my God, this chai is so good."

Then, as Alena pulled into traffic, I encouraged her to continue her story.

"Anyway," she said, glancing at me, "he's really wonderful. He has a son Rowan's age, and we all went to this lake together and everyone got along great. Right, Rowan? Wasn't it fun to go to the lake with Jude and Zack?"

"Yeah, it was," he said with his mouth full of brownie.

"So, what's this new guy's name? Jude?"

She laughed, "No, that's his five-year-old son. He's just six months younger than Rowan. His name is Zack. The new guy I'm dating is Zack."

◆　◆　◆

Alena went on talking about this new man in her life and how well they got along.

"So, anyway, I'd like you and Dad to meet him. I want to introduce him to my friends, too."

"That sounds good."

"So, would it be okay if Zack and Jude flew out here at the end of the week?"

"Here? You mean to Seattle.?"

"Yes, and stay at the house?" Alena's shoulders were beginning to hunch. "Please, please, please?" This obviously meant a lot to her.

"Where would they sleep?"

"In the spare bedroom. I'd organize all the toys. And junk"

"Okay, I guess."

"Oh, that's great," she said, her face glowing.

How could I have said yes! How was I going to do all of this? I was using a walker. And I was so tired.

On the way home, Alena talked more about Zack, explaining that he was a little younger than she was and that he lived in Omaha. He worked as a political consultant and had full custody of Jude.

"You'll really like him," she said. "I'm going to text him as soon as I get to the house so he can make plane reservations."

When we got to the driveway, she was still talking about Zack.. I sipped my chai and tried to be enthusiastic. "I'm looking forward to this," I said. But was I?

◆　◆　◆

Later that afternoon, Alena took Rowan to Green Lake to play on a huge jungle gym and in a sandpit. I was sorry I couldn't go with them—Rowan loved this park—but I think I wouldn't have made it out of the parking lot!

After they had gone, I stood on my deck, breathing in the fresh crisp air and feeling the breeze on my face. I was too nervous to sit on the wrought iron chairs by the picnic table. How would I even get up? So, I just stood there, watching the maple leaves drift down in the backyard. It felt as if I had missed the whole summer. The autumn leaves were starting to pile up. And who was going to rake those leaves this year? That was something I usually did.

Feeling tired, I sat on my couch cushions and drifted off to sleep.

Then, there was a bang, and I woke up with a start. What was that? Had I been dreaming?

I heard something creak, then there was a *knock, knock, knock* at the front door.

"Just a moment," I yelled.

I pushed my fists down on the pillows and stood up. Grabbing my walker, I slowly shuffled to my front window and looked down. A petite middle-aged woman with brown curly hair stood at the front door. I slid the window open.

"Hello?" I called down.

The woman looked up at me and said, "I'm Sarah, the public health nurse." She paused. "Are you Susan?"

"Oh my gosh, I forgot we have an appointment. Please come in. The door is open."

She came upstairs, and I apologized again for forgetting.

"That's okay," she said, "I'm here to check your vitals and see how you're adjusting to being home."

After she took my blood pressure and pulse, she asked me, "Are you here by yourself?"

"Oh no, my daughter is here with my six-year-old grandson for a week. They've gone to play in a park for a little bit."

"I imagine a six-year-old needs to get outside."

"Yes, I guess that's true."

Sarah looked at her clipboard and told me, "I have here that Medicare will be sending a new walker. It will have a seat to sit on or perhaps put a dish on, if you want."

"Really? That's great. It's hard to carry a cup of tea and push this old, borrowed walker."

After we talked for a few minutes, she began to put away her blood pressure cuff and pulse oximeter. She asked, "Are there any questions you have?"

"Well. . .um. . .yes," I said. I didn't quite know how to put this. "My daughter doesn't. . .I mean hasn't been getting home, usually, until after dark. And when I sit here and watch the sky darken, I get this sort of, haunted feeling."

"Uh-huh." She obviously wanted me to say more.

"It's hard to explain," I said, "but it's kind of like. . . well, another day has passed. The day is gone, and it's never to come back. Now it's dark. And then I worry what will happen in the night. Will I even see another morning?"

Her eyes softened. "That's not an unusual feeling to have," she said.

"Really?"

"A lot of people who've been through something traumatic feel this way."

"I don't feel as if I've been through something that's so bad. But I guess I have. After all, I went to my meditation center one evening at the end of July, and then I didn't come back for eight weeks."

She looked puzzled, so I explained. "Last summer I went to our meditation center all dressed up and looking forward to a special evening. When I was there, I started talking weird and this friend, who happened to be a nurse, took me to the ER. They put me in the hospital, and I didn't come home until last week."

"Yes," she said. "That was a long time. So, you went through a lot."

She zipped up her bag, stood and pulled on her sweater. "I'm glad we were able to talk about what you're feeling," she told me.

"Thank you. It really helps to know that it's normal to feel some fear."

◆　◆　◆

A little later, as the sun began to set, I took some pillows from the couch out to the deck, setting them up on one of the chairs and plunking myself down. From that perch, I looked at the sky and watched the crows flying over, calling to each other as they headed to their roosting spot at the UW campus in Bothell. The sky gradually turned pink and then gold. Evening was coming, and what I thought was that soon Rowan would be running up the stairs and telling me all that they had done that afternoon. I felt at peace.

The next morning, I asked Alena if she'd take me to Green Lake.

I told her, "I think if you drop me off in the parking lot, I can make my way down the sidewalk and sit on one of the benches. And it will be so good just to look at the lake."

Alena seemed doubtful, but she agreed to it.

At first, I was nervous about being dropped off while Alena looked for parking. I didn't know how long I'd have to wait for her. What if there was no place to sit while she drove up and down the streets looking for parking? I was worried about walking down the long sidewalk to the lake with no one there. What if I fell? Happily, Alena found a parking place in the main lot.

"You have good parking karma," I said.

She said nothing in response. She opened the car door and placed my walker as close as she could get to the passenger side of the car. I boosted myself up and grabbed onto it.

She seemed sullen, and I didn't understand why. Then I looked at the long sidewalk down to one of the benches by the lake, and my shoulders tensed, my stomach felt tight. How was I actually going to do this? But the bench was empty, and if I could just get to it, I could sit down there and rest for a minute.

I faced myself toward the lake and started walking in that direction.

"Come on, Meemaw," Rowan said, grinning. "You can make it."

"Okay, Rowan," I told him. "Let's get down there before someone else sits on that bench!"

"I'll beat you," he said, beginning to run.

"I bet you will," I said. But I was laughing.

A light breeze blew as I, step-by-step, rolled toward the lake. The lake, sparkling with sunlight, got closer and closer. Finally, I touched the empty bench with my hand.

"I made it," I said triumphantly.

"But I was first!" Rowan said.

"Yes, you certainly were."

I plopped down and looked at the sun reflecting on the lake. It was so good to be doing something normal with Rowan. We both loved coming to Green Lake to watch the ducks and have a treat— and the snack stand was open all year.

Rowan asked if he could go wading, and Alena told him it would be fine, but just up his ankles, and he had to take off his shoes and socks first.

"But before you do," I said to my grandson, "first, sit down by me and let your mom take a picture of us."

Later, I looked at the photo of Rowan and me on my phone. I was sitting with my arm around Rowan and we both had happy smiles on our faces. I had made it down to the beach. It took a lot of energy. I was proud of myself.

Still, I felt tendrils of fear in my body. What if this was as much as I could ever do? What if I never walked around Green Lake again?

Chapter 25

WHEN GUESTS COME

I gazed out my sliding glass door at the bright October day. Most of the Norway maple leaves had turned from bright green to copper and were lying on the mossy grass. The sweetgum's vibrant yellow leaves hung valiantly onto the branches and shimmered in the sunlight. Early that morning, Mary Lou had picked up Alena and Rowan and taken them to the airport to welcome Zack and Jude.

They left me at home. If I'd been able to get up off the couch, I could have gone outside for a while. I wanted to sit in the sun and breathe in the sharp, cold air, fragrant with the smell of leaves and the fallen fruit of my neighbor's apple tree. It was frustrating that I didn't have enough energy even to open the door—let alone sit down on the deck and get up again later!

In the kitchen, I saw the round aluminum teapot sitting on my stove and thought that a cup of English Breakfast tea would be nice—but then I wondered how I would get that cup of tea back to the coffee table.

I considered the fancy, red walker that Medicare had just provided. It had a fold-down seat I could use if a chair wasn't available—and that I could use to transport a cup of tea as well. But first I had to get up from the couch. The two pillows beneath me were smashed down far into the cushion. It would probably be safest to just sit here and read until everyone got back from the airport.

I opened to the second chapter of the murder mystery I'd been plowing through. Setting the book down, I sighed. I didn't feel like reading a mystery right now, and it was going to be a while before everyone got back. After they picked up Zack and his son, Alena was taking them all out to lunch. That would be a couple of hours at least.

I wanted to go out to lunch myself. Well, at least I could make myself some tea.

Gathering my courage, I scooted forward on the pillows. I caught hold of the walker handles, but the walker rolled forward just enough to put getting up off the couch out of my reach.

"Damn it!"

William woke up at that and looked at me with wide green eyes. He still wouldn't sit on my lap. He spent his time on the recliner. Even so, he was good company.

"I'm going to do this, William," I said. Then I counted, "One. . .two. . .three."

I pushed my fists down into the pillows and raised myself up high enough that I could take hold of the walker handles. I squeezed on the hand brake before the walker could roll too much.

"I did it," I sang out. "I did it! William, I did it!"

The cat was apparently unimpressed. He buried his head in his paws.

◆　◆　◆

I made my celebratory cup of tea and maneuvered it back to the couch, spilling about a quarter of the liquid onto the walker's seat.

"Maybe not so full next time, Susan," I told myself. But then there was another challenge: how was I going to sit down on the couch while holding a hot cup of tea?

After a few moments pondering this, it finally occurred to me to set the tea on the coffee table within reaching distance of the couch and then use the walker to sit back down.

That managed, I sat on the couch, reading my book and enjoying the treat I had managed to get for myself. It was lovely.

A couple of hours later, the front door opened, and two pairs of feet came running to the top of the stairs.

"Hi Meemaw, this is Jude," Rowan called out as he ran down the hall.

A smiling little boy with brown curly hair waved at me while galloping after my grandson.

"Well, hi Jude," I shouted. "Have fun with the toys."

Alena smiled at the boys as they ran down the hall.

"I guess that's Jude," I said.

"Yes, that's Jude. And this is his dad, Zack." A dark-haired young man walked into the living room, his face lit by a sweet smile. Alena said to him, "This is my mom, Susan."

"Hi Susan," Zack said. "It's very nice to meet you."

"Can I offer you a cup of tea?"

"Sure."

"I'll make it, Mom," Alena said.

"Oh, yeah, it takes me awhile."

Zack and I talked while Alena made the tea and then tidied her bedroom. I had been wondering about the sleeping arrangements. Were Alena and Zack sleeping together? Alena's old bedroom and mine were directly across from each other, and I still could remember her giggles coming through the walls in the middle of the night while she talked on and on with boyfriends. I finally decided that I didn't care who slept with whom as long as they were quiet at night.

"So, I understand you were a like a free-lance political consultant. What does that involve?" I asked, focusing on Zack.

"Well, sometimes I'm hired to work on getting state initiatives passed, like, say, the revocation of the death penalty in the state. Or I might work on getting a state legislator reelected."

"And also, Mom," Alena said, popping back into the living room, "Zack was the director of the 2012 campaign for Obama in Nebraska."

"Wow!"

"Yeah, the youngest campaign manager ever."

"How old were you?" I asked him.

"Twenty-three."

"That's impressive."

"Guess what?" Jude said, running into the room.

"What?" I said.

"This was the first time I've ever been on an airplane."

"That is so cool. Was it exciting?"

"Yeah, and when I looked out the windows, I could see the *mountains* way below us."

"And you had to tell everyone in the plane that this was your first time flying, huh," Zack said.

"Jude, come on, let's keep on playing," Rowan yelled.

"Oka-a-ay, but I'm the bad guy this time," he hollered, running back into Rowan's room.

"Well, I better get our air bed blown up," Zack said. "It was nice talking to you."

"You, too." I leaned back against the couch and relaxed for a minute.

Alena was happier than I'd seen her in a long time. And Zack is really bright and engaging. I might just like this guy.

♦ ♦ ♦

The next day after breakfast, the smell of eggs and coffee lingered in the air. The late morning sun streamed in the window, capturing the floating dust motes.

"Thank you, once again, for the good breakfast, Sweetie," I said to Alena.

"You're welcome, Mumsie. I'm going to vacuum and then we'll be taking off."

"I imagine you'll be gone until late," I said, trying to keep the hint of disappointment from my voice.

"Of course, we will, Mom. I want Dad to meet Zack, and that's about a two-hour drive one direction over the pass. And we'll probably stop at Snoqualmie Falls on the way back."

A little later, as they backed out of the driveway, I felt my throat tighten and blinked back tears, glad that no one could see me.

What was I going to do with myself the rest of the day? I could practice my physical therapy exercises—cross your arms around your chest; stand up; sit down.

I tried but could only manage a couple of times, and that was with using my arms to boost myself up. My legs were still too weak.

Feeling listless, I stared out the living room window hoping to catch Diane in her yard with her Husky, Tui. They weren't outside.

My eyelids grew heavy, and I drifted off to sleep. Sometime later my phone rang. It was Lily.

"Hi Mom. How's it going?"

"Hi Lily. It's so good to hear your voice! It's going okay, I guess."

"That doesn't sound so good. Aren't you feeling good?"

"I'm kind of tired. Jude and Rowan start running up and down the hall at six in the morning."

"Wow, that's early."

"I talked to Alena this morning, and Zack said he'd keep Jude in bed until seven—so that's a little better."

"What have you guys been doing?"

"Alena's been showing Zack around Seattle every day, and today they went over to Cle Elum to see your dad. They're gone every day.

"*Hmm.*"

"They leave me by myself," I said, wiping the tears from my face.

"Oh, Mom. It's just not right to leave you alone so much."

"I know."

"Well, I'll cook you a lot of nice meals starting next Monday. It's just a few days. Will you be okay until then?"

"Yes. I'm sorry for breaking down. I don't know why I've been so emotional. Alena does leave me food, of course. She's just all involved with Zack."

"She really likes him, Mom, and after what she's been through, that's good."

"I know."

"And this is her last week of vacation time. She used a lot of days when she was in the hospital with you."

"Yeah, that's right. It's so weird that I don't have any memory of that."

"She might be thinking of this week as a vacation. But, like I said, I'll be there soon."

"Okay, I'm looking forward to it. We can eat lots of desserts and watch Dr. Phil, like we used to."

"Yeah," Lily said, laughing.

◆ ◆ ◆

The next morning Alena told me she wanted to show Zack and Jude the Space Needle.

"Oh, that's great!" I said. "What time are we going? I need to get ready. It takes me a while to navigate the shower bench and stuff."

"Mom, we can't take you. It would be too much."

"What do you mean? Can't you just drop me off where the cars pull in by the Space Needle? You know, like you did for Mother's Day that one year," I said, sounding like a puppy begging for attention.

"It just won't work," she said, shaking her head.

"But we talked about showing Zack the Space Needle, and Seattle Center. We talked about it. Don't you remember?" My voice was quivering.

"You always do this, Mom. You just go crazy. Why do you have to be this way?"

I stared at her speechless. I didn't want to cry so I tipped my head back slightly hoping the tears would somehow roll back into my eyes.

We *had* talked about it! We had talked about showing Zack and Jude the Seattle Center. Alena knew that this is one of my favorite places.

Rowan ran into the living room breaking the tension. In a little while, they all left for another day's adventure.

After they left, my heart felt heavy until my downstairs tenant knocked on the door and came up to visit for a while. She offered to do my laundry and pick up anything I needed at the grocery store.

Later, my brother called and made plans to come and visit.

Everyone was being so nice. Maybe I was expecting too much of Alena.

◆　◆　◆

Early Saturday morning, I lay in bed and listened to Alena and Zack get the kids out the door to catch a shuttle to the airport. The night before, they'd offered to take me to Fremont to see the sights, but I was concerned about being able to walk up the hills, so at the last minute, I backed out.

We had all gone out to lunch one afternoon—and that was kind of awkward for everyone. I just didn't get what was going on with Alena. Didn't she realize that I'd been in a hospital and in rehab for eight weeks?

Oh well. She was in love.

It was still dark, and a damp wind was blowing the trees. I pulled my comforter around my shoulders and eased back to sleep.

Chapter 26

WILL YOU BE
THERE FOR ME?

I opened my eyes, and my room came into focus. I looked at my picture of my smiling guru sitting on my dresser. The house was silent except for the rain pattering against the window. My senses attuned to Alena's bedroom.

I rolled over in bed from my back to my side. I could feel the shimmering energy of Alena in her bedroom across the hall.

Was she awake yet? I couldn't hear her. Had she already gone to school? Then Alena's energy dissolved like an echo reverberating on distant canyon walls. Of course, Alena wasn't in her room. She didn't live here anymore.

I sighed and rolled to my back.

No one lived here anymore.

I got annoyed with myself. Enough of this!

◆ ◆ ◆

I threw off my comforter and scooched to the edge of the bed, took hold of my walker, and stood. It was time to start my day. After I'd brushed my teeth, I made my way to the kitchen and put the tea kettle on to boil. I went into the living room and stood looking out at the tulip tree. That tree had been so beautiful in the spring with scores of brilliant pink flowers. Now a few sparse yellow leaves clung to the branches.

Unbidden came the image of the way the tree had looked two years earlier. Then the leaves had blazed like luminous golden jewels scintillating in the sun. The fall colors that year were unsurpassable. In late October that year, I had been looking at the tree from the living room while I listened to Alena and Lily talk during a rare weekend visit together. It had been so sweet to have both my daughters overnight at my house. At the time, I didn't know that they were keeping a secret from me. The memory felt like a stab in my heart. Just then the tea kettle shrieked, and I went to make my tea.

A few minutes later, I pushed my way to the couch, careful not to spill the tea. Had it been only two years?

Just two years ago, Alena and Rowan's father were still married, Rowan was four, and the family was living in Olympia. Alena had been working, but her husband wasn't. He was depressed and drinking too much—and looking for a job. I was worried they'd move to Minnesota to be close to his parents. It would have been easier for him to find work there, but I cried every time Alena talked about it. I couldn't stand the thought of being so far from Rowan.

I'd been there at Rowan's birth, and I was filled with joy when I got to hold him in my arms. I felt like I'd always known Rowan. I would babysit every chance I had, and after a while he began spending the night at my house.

The first night he was upset. He must have been about two. When he realized that his mom wasn't coming to pick him up this time, he announced that he was going to walk home. There he was, dressed in his footie pajamas, heading downstairs to the front door. I told him I'd keep him safe. He eventually settled down and, later, he slept just fine. That was the first of many overnights. He'd played in the park at Green Lake and loved to swim at the huge kid's pool in Mountlake Terrace. Sometimes we'd go to a movie or to Seattle Center to an event or just to play in the International Fountain. I'd loved every minute with my grandson.

Eventually, Alena started talking about buying a house in Olympia and suggested I look for a house nearby. I stopped worrying about them moving.

Then came the phone call.

I was lying on my bed deep in meditation. My meditations were usually peaceful and velvety dark. This time an image floated before me. It was Rowan standing on the lawn at the park that sloped gently down to Green Lake. The sky was pewter gray, and Rowan had his plaid green coat on. His hands were in fists by his sides, like they were cold. His short blond hair ruffled in the wind. He looked at me with sorrowful eyes and said something I couldn't quite understand.

"What did you say?" I asked.

"Meemaw, will you. . ." His voice faded into the wind.

"What, Rowan? What are you saying?"

For a moment I was distracted by the sun emerging from the clouds, lighting up the lake with twinkling diamond-shaped sparkles.

"Meemaw!" he called, his voice becoming urgent.

"What, Rowan, Sweetie? What are you trying to say?"

"Will you be there for me?" He came closer now and looked up at me. He seemed so small and alone.

"Will I be there for you? Well, yes, I'll be there for as long as I can," I answered thinking I probably would be alive through his high school years, at least.

"Will you, Meemaw?"

"Of course." I turned and looked at the silvery light that was shimmering even brighter on the water. "But I first I have to. . ."

I didn't finish my sentence. I was so drawn to that light. Was I supposed to walk into the light?

I opened my eyes then; I was looking at the ceiling. What a meditation! This was the second time I'd had a vision of Rowan standing at Green Lake, asking me if I'd be there for him.

I checked my phone and saw that there were several calls from Alena. I snuffed out the candle and called her back.

"Mom, I've been trying to get hold of you! Where have you been?"

"Meditating. I had the phone turned off. Is everything all right?"

"Are you sitting down? I have something to tell you."

"You're pregnant," I said, smiling.

She laughed. "No, I'm not pregnant." She didn't say anything more.

"Alena, you're making me nervous. What's going on?"

"We're moving."

"Oh!" I'd felt like I'd been punched in the stomach.

"Mom?"

"Why?"

"Ken got a full-time job, a permanent government contract."

"Okay, where?" I was hoping it was close to Seattle.

"Lincoln, Nebraska."

"Nebraska?" That was not close to Seattle! It was that flat brown land I've seen on flights across the country!

"Yes, and housing is so cheap there we can buy a house!"

"Oh, I see. My voice had gone flat, but I tried to sound supportive. "That's good."

"And I can stay home with Rowan."

"I guess you've always wanted to be at home with him. When are you leaving?"

"Three weeks."

"Three weeks!"

"Yes, I was so scared I didn't tell you right away, but you're taking this so much better than I'd thought you would. I was afraid you'd burst into tears."

"So, you've known for a while."

"Yes. We found out the middle of October."

"Oh. Did Lily know?"

"I told her when we stayed together at your house."

Ice water began running through my veins. I could barely process what she was saying. Right now was the second week in November, so there would be no Thanksgiving or Christmas together. No more overnights with Rowan for God knew how long.

♦ ♦ ♦

The day before they left, I drove to Olympia to say goodbye. The movers were in the midst of packing everything. Ken was supervising, and Alena was at the vet with the cat. I sat in their master bedroom on the queen-sized bed with Rowan so we could be out of everyone's way. Rowan wanted to play, but the only thing available was a penny and a paper clip. I felt so heavy with sadness that after a short time my imagination ran dry.

"Rowan, I have to leave now."

"But who am I going to play with?" he asked, his voice growing desperate.

"I don't know, Sweetie. But your mom will be home soon. Remember, Rowan. . ."

"I know, never give up," he said with a slight smile.

"Never give up."

I hugged him and said goodbye. I drove home fighting tears all the way.

The winter after they'd moved, I'd felt like someone had died. My friends and family didn't understand. No one *had* died, after all. People would say things like, "You'll see them again." They'd say things like, "Of course, you love Rowan, but he isn't the source of love. Love lies inside you." My mind knew they were right, but that's not how my body experienced it. I had continual back pain and lost over fifteen pounds. I sat by the window every morning listening to the Oregon juncos trilling their sad song and reading a book on how to be fearless.

Time passed. I visited Lincoln every four or five months, and when I was home, I spent time seeing friends and relatives, and volunteering at the meditation center. Eventually, the sadness lifted.

A crow cawed loudly, bringing me back to the present. I finished drinking my lukewarm tea and stared at the tulip tree with its sad yellow leaves. I'd hated that tree for a long time. I felt that its beauty was mocking me with the painful secret that Alena had kept from me that October weekend two years before.

Of course, it wasn't the tree's fault that my daughter hadn't had the courage to tell me she was moving. And I did love the tree's pink blossoms in the spring.

I took a deep breath in and tried to exhale the sadness I was feeling. I realized that I would have moved to Nebraska in a second. But now Alena had a new love; she didn't want her mother nearby.

I went into the kitchen and looked at the stack of papers on my counter. I picked up a pile and spotted a bright blue pamphlet with the bracing title: "Should I Put My Parent in Continuing Care? Options for Families."

What the hell was this? Were my daughters planning to park me in a nursing home? What was going on? I covered my face with my hands—but for just a moment.

I couldn't think about this now. I'd ask Lily about it when she got here tomorrow.

Chapter 27

A NEAR-FATAL ENCOUNTER

It was pouring rain when Lily arrived the next morning. The fir trees were dripping, and water was backing up in the street from the overtaxed storm drain grates. Mary Lou dropped Lily off and waved at me as she backed out of the driveway.

"Hi, Mum," Lily said, enfolding me in her arms. "It's so good to see you."

"Oh, you poor honey," I said, stroking her long, wet hair. "You're drenched. I'm glad you're here safe and sound. I was worried about Mary Lou driving you in her little car."

"She took Martin Luther King most of the way, which is only twenty-five miles an hour, so no worries. It's sure good to see you up and around," she said, eyeing my walker.

"Yeah, I'm doing okay. Sit down. I'll make you some tea." Now, I could make the tea!

I put the kettle on to boil, and my heart was filled with happiness. "I haven't seen you in so long," I said.

"For sure. But I did spend a lot of time in the hospital with you, remember?"

"Not really," I told her. "I do have a vague recollection of begging you to give me the keys to my car so I could drive home. You said, 'no way' and got really irritated with me."

I could picture us sitting in the expansive hospital restaurant overlooking the Sound. It occurred to me in that moment that it was sort of strange that the restaurant had been on the same level as the water. It seemed as though they might be concerned about flooding.

"You were in no way ready to go home."

"I do remember when I woke up right before I was supposed to get an MRI and said, 'Hi Lily.' Everyone started laughing and clapping, right?"

"Yeah, we were all stunned. You had been so out of it."

"What I remember is that I was so excited to tell you about this vivid dream I'd had right before I woke up. It was very scary. I thought I was going to disintegrate into little pieces. It was such a dramatic experience, and then to come out of it and find you standing there! I was trying to tell you about it when you were wheeling me back to my room."

"You may not realize it, Mom, but you really weren't making much sense."

"I just wanted to make sure that you understood that I finally recognized you on that stage and the love I felt drew me back to reality."

Lily twisted her long auburn hair around on her index finger and looked out of the window. She seemed anxious.

"Are you tired, Sweetie?" I asked, handing her the cup of tea.

"I had to get to the airport really early today, so, yeah, I'm kind of tired."

"Did Matt take you?"

"Hardly," she scoffed. "He stayed up all night playing video games," she said, checking her phone. "I haven't heard from him even though I've messaged him about five times. Do you think I should call him?"

I sighed. This is the way it had always been with Lily and her boyfriends. She was always contacting them. Lily was such a great person. I had never understood why she needed so much reassurance.

What I said was, "I don't know, Sweetie. Maybe."

"I think I will. And then I'll sit down and drink my tea."

She went to the guest bedroom to make the call. I heard her talking from there. Well, anyway, at least she'd reached him. That was a relief. A few minutes later she came in frowning. I asked her if everything was okay.

"Oh, he's really down. He gets so depressed that it makes me worry. Vets have such high rates of suicide, especially in Montana."

"Has he threatened suicide?"

"Suicide by cop."

"What does that mean?"

"If I call the cops, he'll point a gun at them, and then they'd eventually shoot him."

"Oh my God! But why would you call the cops?"

"Mom, I don't want to talk about it right now. I think I'll call his vet friends and see if one of them can stop by and check on him."

I said, "Good idea," but what I thought was that she should tell his friends not to bring any booze with them. Alcohol was the last thing Matt needed right now.

On one of my visits, I'd witnessed a blowout fight between Matt and Lily at a time when they'd both been drinking. I found it frightening. I'd wanted to go back to my hotel, but I stayed with them in case my daughter needed protection. Matt was big and strong, and he could easily have overpowered Lily.

I massaged my eyebrows with my thumb and fingers. I didn't want to be thinking about this right now. I just wanted to enjoy Lily's visit.

◆　◆　◆

We managed to relax for a while and chat about family and what foods I'd like to eat. Then Lily, grocery list in hand, headed for Central Market.

"Don't forget cheesecake!" I called out to her as she left.

As soon as I was alone, I made my way back to my bedroom to catch a nap. It was amazing how tired I was every day.

I put the mantra on and glided into sleep.

A little later I felt a gentle pat on my bottom and opened my eyes to see a smiling Lily sitting on the edge of my bed.

"That's how my mom used to wake me every morning for high school," I said, my heart warming with the memory. Tears formed in my eyes. I missed my mother.

"Are you okay, Mom?"

I told her I was fine—and that I didn't know why I was so sensitive lately.

"You've been through a lot," she said. "Why don't I cut you some cheesecake."

"That sounds good. What kind did you get?"

"The kind with six different flavors."

"My favorite."

Later, I took my plate to the kitchen and saw another bright blue pamphlet with the title about continuing care.

"Lily, what exactly is this?" I asked, waving the brochure at her. "Are you thinking of putting me in a nursing home?"

Lily had a little edge to her voice as she answered: "For a while when you were in the hospital, we didn't know what you would be like when you woke up—or even *if* you'd wake up."

It was the edge I responded to. I said, "Why are you so irritated with me right now? Did I give you a too hard time at the hospital?"

"I'm not irritated with you. It was scary, though. No one seemed to know what was wrong with you and whether you were going to wake up at all. And then when you did come around, it was apparent that you had a long way to go before you could be on your own."

I sat down on the couch across from her. Lily was in the easy chair with William sitting in her lap. She stroked the cat as we talked.

I told her, "I remember when we were in the restaurant, I insisted you drive me home or at least give me the car keys so I could drive myself."

Lily was quiet for a moment, and then she looked at me curiously. "What restaurant?" she asked.

"You know the one on the bottom floor of the hospital."

"What are you talking about?" She arched an eyebrow, looking at me quizzically.

"The really pretty one with the big glass windows overlooking the Sound. Nadine was there too. The doctors came down, and she asked them some questions."

"Mom, I hate to tell you this, but there's no restaurant like that in Virginia Mason."

My head started to swim. "No?"

"No! You never left your hospital rooms except to take medical tests."

"Really. But. . ." Was it possible I had imagined all of this? I didn't put that thought into words, but Lily addressed it for me.

She said, "You were probably hallucinating."

I didn't know how to respond. The memory was so vivid to me. I could even smell the coffee being poured. Could I have had the same hallucination twice? It was beginning to seem likely that I had.

Finally, I said, "I guess I wouldn't have been sitting in a fancy restaurant wearing my hospital gown and with my hair sticking up all over the place."

Lily laughed. "No," she said. "But at least it was a pleasant hallucination!"

"You know when I was begging you to take me home, I could see my house in my mind's eye."

"Oh yeah?"

"And you know what? It didn't look like my house at all. It was little and white and sitting with a sloping driveway beside it, and in front of the property was a rockery for flowers and succulents. I wonder how I even imagined that?"

"I don't know," Lily said. "Your brain was in a weird place."

That night in bed I stared at the ceiling listening to the guru chant. I started wondering just how much of what I remembered from the hospital had actually happened. How much didn't happen? And what did happen that I didn't remember?

I could remember the many different rooms I'd been put in. Sometimes I'd wake up to a brand new one, and sometimes it seemed familiar, like when I was in the professor's office.

Then it occurred to me—why would I ever, ever be in a professor's office at the hospital! Why would I be seeing the other "dorms" from my room—with the sunlight glinting off the windows. I remembered being grateful that I'd been loaned this room to stay in.

None of that was true. I felt like I'd been watching a movie where I assumed one plot line and then encountered a twist that meant everything I thought was true wasn't.

I groaned. Maybe my brain was still messed up.

♦ ♦ ♦

As the week passed, Lily and I both relaxed. Lily enjoyed making me meals, and we had plenty of time to eat good food and watch entertaining TV. The day before Lily was scheduled to leave, I went to see my rheumatologist for the first time since I'd come home from my eight-week ordeal. I needed to check in with her and obtain a doctor's statement to claim travel insurance benefits so I could be reimbursed for canceling my trip to India.

The doctor greeted me with a brilliant smile. A petite woman of Indian descent, she is always patient with me and thorough in answering my questions.

"How are you, Susan?"

I told her that I was glad to be here and in one piece.

"Yes, you've been through a lot," she said. She checked on how my new medication was working. I asked her about the weakness I was experiencing in my legs.

"It could be the inactivity, but it's probably because of your poor brain."

"That's kind of scary. But at least I didn't have brain cancer," I said with a nervous laugh.

Afterward, as I took the elevator down to the first floor, I read the short note the doctor had written to the insurance company:

Susan Bruzas must miss the trip to India because she will need a great deal of time to recover from a near-fatal encounter with viral encephalitis.

What did the doctor mean by "near-fatal encounter"? Had I really been that sick? Maybe she just wanted to make sure I got my money back? I didn't almost die!

Did I?

Chapter 28

THE WIND WHIPPED THE TREES AROUND ME

"**S**usie Minoozie! How are you?"

I always laughed when my little sister called me that funny name. A long time ago, when we were in our twenties, I had gone to a party at her house. We all got fairly inebriated, and her friend started calling me Susie Minoozie. The name stuck.

"I'm getting better and better, Nadinie. Lily took good care of me."

"How's the therapy going?"

"There's a really good physical therapist coming over twice a week, and she has me doing exercises to strengthen my legs. I can get around with my walker pretty well."

I didn't articulate my fear that I might not be able to ever graduate to walking without assistance. And I wasn't telling anyone what my doctor had said about it being my "poor brain" that had caused my legs to be so weak. My friends and family had been through enough with me. I was determined to walk again without a walker or cane!

We talked for a while longer before I got to the reason I had called.

"Nadine, I want to ask you a strange question."

"Ye-e-es?"

I told her about my realization during a conversation with Lily that there had been no plush restaurant at the hospital—even though that restaurant figured largely in my experience at the time.

"So, I remember being in the same place with you!" I finished.

"You're kidding!" she said

I told her how the restaurant had looked to me and how several doctors had come in to talk with her while we were there. I asked her if she remembered any doctors coming into my room while she was with me—one who did my brain biopsy and another who was an infectious disease specialist.

Nadine did remember the doctors. So, meeting and talking with the doctors had actually happened. Except—as I clarified with Nadine—it had happened in my hospital room.

"I must have really, *really* wanted to get out of that room," I said.

"Yeah," Nadine said. "And it's kind of weird and scary that you're just now realizing there was no beautiful restaurant."

I decided to put a better spin on this. "It wasn't really an unpleasant mirage," I pointed out. "I must have associated you and Lily with elegance, beauty, and good things!"

She laughed. "Do you remember telling me and the speech therapist that Virginia Mason had rooms in the parking lot of a shopping center, and you'd spent the night in the back seat of a car?"

A vague memory came to me of darkness, rain, and the gray back seat of a car. Then came the image of white scratchy mittens tied to my wrists.

"Oh my God, yes. I do remember the vivid experience of being in the back seat of a car." I paused. "And I also remember how you and that lady sitting next to you looked at each other when I woke up and told you that there were hospital rooms in the parking lot of Fred Meyer. I could tell you didn't believe me."

"She was the speech therapist, and she'd just told me that you were still having some processing problems."

"So, my telling you I'd spent the night in a room that just happened to be in a parking lot was a perfect illustration of that!"

We both laughed. Still, I was cringing with embarrassment. I felt like a child who'd been caught in a lie.

After talking for a few minutes longer, Nadine rang off.

◆　◆　◆

I sat on the couch staring at the grey clouds sailing across the sky and pondering all of this. Of course, when I was in the hospital, I'd never been sleeping in the back seat of the car or eating at a fancy restaurant. How many other places had I imagined?

A deep unease began to seep through me like frigid glacial water. I felt chilled and drained of energy, pulled my comforter around me, and closed my eyes for a few minutes but couldn't relax.

Why couldn't I remember large swaths of time, especially after the brain biopsy? Where had I been during that time? And when I finally started remembering, why did I still think I'd spent the night in a Fred Meyer parking lot?

I decided to look at the paperwork from the hospital. I thought I'd seen a discharge summary written by the doctor. Maybe that would give me some clues. Without too much trouble, I boosted myself up from the sofa and went into the kitchen with the aid of my walker. As my upper body got stronger, I was having an easier time getting around. On the kitchen counter, inside a glossy folder emblazoned with the name Virginia Mason Medical Center, I found a discharge summary written by Dr. H dated September 6, 2015.

Under diagnosis/discharge, I read this:

Encephalopathy with meningoencephalitis and leptomeningeal enhancing lesions and hemorrhage, etiology is unknown, clinically resolving, much improved.

What the heck did any of that mean?

I started looking up definitions for the labels the doctor had written and jotted them down right on the discharge paper. When I read over what I'd written, my chest became so constricted I could barely breathe.

A very serious neurological condition resembling both meningitis and encephalitis. An infection of the meninges, the membranes that surround the brain and spinal cord. A serious condition affecting the brain that requires prompt treatment to lower the risk of lasting complication or death. The recovery process may take months to even years. Survivors of severe cases can be left with permanent problems.

Requires prompt treatment to lower the risk of lasting complication or death. That was the statement that jumped out at me. I definitely had not been treated promptly. At first, they'd thought I had metastatic brain cancer. They did a spinal tap on me that first week. I do remember that.

I put the papers back in the folder and sat staring out of the window at a mist in my yard. Behind the mist, I could see the bare snowball bush and the Japanese Maple. Perhaps the mist was beginning to lift on my brain as well. I was feeling sharper than I had felt before, but I still had so many questions. Where had my soul been during the two weeks between the biopsy and when I woke up on the MRI table and saw Lily? Where was the consciousness I think of as "me"?

◆　◆　◆

That night, I finally got William to cuddle with me in bed. Enjoying the closeness of the cat's warmth, I thought again about what I had just been through. I'd had a rare disease that the doctors had trouble diagnosing correctly. Their assessment had been that either I would die or I would be so impaired I would have to spend the rest of my life in residential long-term care. Against daunting odds, I had come back—from not being able to swallow, coherently speak, walk, pee by myself and also from hallucinations that I was sitting in a car or a restaurant or God only knew where else.

My doctors had been saying that this was a miracle cure, but after all that I'd been through, was there some kind of emotional trauma buried deep within me?

I listened to the rain pattering against my window and pulled the comforter under my chin and drifted off to sleep.

♦   ♦   ♦

I opened my eyes, jarred awake. I was sitting on something wet. Where was I?

I looked around, trying to see through a murky darkness. I was able to make out some concrete steps and a railing—it was the steps that led up to my front door. Oh my God! I was sitting in in my front yard, on the grass in front of my house.

My heart thrummed hard, and my breathing became rapid.

How had I gotten here?—outside! Down the stairs! Had I walked in my sleep? I used to do that, as a child. Had I done it again?

The night was starless, and the wind whipped the trees around me as I turned over onto all fours and pushed myself up off the rocky ground.

I had to get back inside my house. I had to get back to my bed. How was I going to do that?

I walked a few steps, grabbed the railing, and pulled myself up the front steps, praying that the front door wouldn't be locked. I turned the knob and pushed. Thank God, it opened. Now, I was going to have to climb the long stairway. Were my legs strong enough?

Step-by-step, I pulled myself up to the landing. A shadowy dark-ness pervaded my house. I looked down the inky black hallway, and my warm, safe bed seemed so far away. How would I ever get there? My bedroom was straight down the hallway, but I knew that I would feel better with a little light.

I reached my arm out and touched the wall. I walked a few steps, letting my hand guide me. When I got to the light switch, I pushed it up. Nothing happened. I tried several more times, but still there was no light.

I wondered if there was someone else in the house—someone who had gone down to the basement and cut the power!

I stood for a moment longer until I realized that I had been through this before. I was dreaming. I'd had this dream before. I knew that I had to get the light to come on before I would wake up. I couldn't seem to get the hall light to come on, but maybe I could turn on the light by my bed.

Taking slow, sure steps and tracking the wall with my right hand, I visualized the small Tiffany table lamp that stood by my bed. The lamp had been my mother's, and the shade had leaded glass pieces shaped like green leaves and orange lotus flowers growing out of turquoise water.

I had never had my consciousness travel this far from my sleeping body. I felt that I wouldn't be able to wake up unless I managed to get back to my sleeping form. So, I set off walking toward my bedroom, repeating my mantra with each step.

After what seemed like hours, I could finally feel the smooth wood of the bedstead against my hand. I sat on the mattress and pulled down on the lamp chain. The light came on, and immediately I woke up. I was lying in my bed.

The bedroom was still dark, but ambient light seeped in from under the window shade and, unlike the total silence of my nightmare, I could hear the sounds of distant traffic.

But was I truly awake?

Tentatively, I reached across to the lamp and pulled down on the chain. The light came on.

That was the sign: I was awake. I was still vibrating with fear, and I took several deep, restorative breaths.

I tossed and turned a bit, and then I threw off the blankets and took hold of my cane. I was strong enough to walk into the living room using just the cane for support. I stood at the living room window for a few minutes and looked at the waning moon illuminating the yard with pools of silvery light. It was a quiet night. There was no wind, and I felt as if I could hear everyone in the neighborhood breathing in and out as they peacefully slept. I sat down on the couch, and William jumped onto my lap. Stroking his fur, I thought about my nightmare.

Did it have anything to do with the trauma of being so sick? I didn't remember anything at all that happened in the two weeks following my biopsy. Was a part of me desperate to awaken my memory? Was part of me wanting just to move on?

At one point in my life, lucid dreaming had been entertaining. It had been fun. I'd open my eyes in my darkened bedroom and actually sit up and look around. To make sure I was dreaming I'd see if my fingers could go through the wall. They always did. I'd fly out the window and around the darkened neighborhood, and sometimes I'd fly straight up into the sky as far as I could go. Whenever I was in a situation where something was chasing me, I would backflip and fall into another dream. It had always been such a great adventure!

But what had happened tonight was not fun at all. The only thing that seemed to save me was repeating my mantra. I needed to remember that.

Chapter 29

CELEBRATION OF LIFE

Later that morning, I took a shower and tried to forget the night before. JoAnne and Louie were driving up from Oregon to stay a few days so they could attend a wedding. Louie was already anxious to help me, so we had a trip to Home Depot planned to select kitchen cabinet knobs for him to put on.

When they got there, we were all giving each other big hugs.

"It's good to see you looking so well, Susie," JoAnne said, holding me at arm's length so she could get a better look.

Louie's arms were already full. He brought in three bags of groceries, one with flowers sticking out of it.

"What's this?" I asked. "You didn't have to bring me groceries. Mary Lou already went shopping for me."

"Well," JoAnne said, smiling. "Earl and Reva are coming down this evening and we are having a belated birthday party for you. I'm making baked chicken."

"You are?" Tears were flooding my eyes. "For me? That's so sweet!"

"Now stop that," JoAnne said. "You're going to make me cry. I'm just so happy you're well."

Soon the table was set with flowers, placemats, fancy napkins, and my favorite green pottery dishes. JoAnne's chicken was simmering in the oven, and Louie had made a huge green salad.

There was a knock, and Louie opened the front door.

"Hey, Bruzas," Earl said, coming up the stairs. "You're looking good!"

"Hi Bro. I guess I got to live. Hi, Reva, it's great to see you too."

"Hi Sis." She set a bag on the kitchen counter.

"Just in time you two," JoAnne said. "Time to eat."

As we passed the food around, I felt joy expand like the sun coming out from behind a dark cloud. I was so fortunate to have this wonderful family who had encouraged me and been there for me through the perils of the last few months.

"When JoAnne and Louie leave, are you going to be able to take care of yourself?" Reva asked me.

"I think I am. I can order food, cook simple meals, drop my laundry bag down the stairs and hold onto the railing to get downstairs to do the washing and drying.

"I think I just heard someone knocking on the door," Reva said.

"Halloo," Mary Lou called up the stairs. "Susan?"

"Mary Lou, come up," I hollered back. "We're having a celebration."

"Oh, wonderful."

"Sit at the other end of the table, Mary Lou," I said. "You deserve a position of honor since you not only helped me, but you helped the kids too, and you made sure I had plenty of visitors."

"Happy birthday to you," Reva sang as she carried the cake in, and everyone joined in, singing loudly and, for the most part, in tune.

"I think this is really a celebration of life party," I said as we ate the delicious cake—a white cake with chocolate icing, my favorite!

"I cried in front of Father Pascal," JoAnne said. "I thought God had deserted me and you. He laughed and said God was still there. And whenever I talked to Earl, he'd tell me, 'Susan will be fine!'"

Earl said, "She'd gotten back on her feet so many times, why not now."

"Were you ever really worried about me?" I asked Mary Lou.

"A little," Mary Lou said, "when they said that you had metastasized brain cancer."

"Hey," Reva interjected, "this is supposed to be a celebration. So, let's be happy."

We all agreed and continued on, recognizing our good fortune that we were all healthy and together.

◆　◆　◆

Rain spattered on the car's windshield as I wound through the Capitol Hill neighborhood with its graceful older homes on my way to the doctor. I was happy that I'd been practicing driving to the grocery stores and Starbucks enough that it now felt safe and natural to make a more complex trip.

Halloween had been a couple of days before. I had really enjoyed seeing the neighborhood kids coming to my door, dressed in ingenious and funny costumes. Their parents had greeted me with amazement, surprised I was able to make it downstairs.

And, of course, I hadn't gone downstairs for each group. I just stayed downstairs, holding onto the railing until the next group came. I was proud of myself for figuring it out.

Now, I was using my cane to get from where I parked to the office of an ear, nose, and throat specialist. I had decided to consult an otolaryngologist about my hoarse voice, which wasn't getting any better.

The doctor was a young woman—I was becoming accustomed to how youthful doctors seemed to me. I gave her a brief summary of my bout with viral encephalitis and my continual scratchy voice. She took a small mirror with a long handle and stuck it down my throat to look at my vocal folds.

She seemed surprised. "There's so much mucous that it's hard to see them."

Trying not to gag kept me from responding.

She had me pronounce vowels—*ah, ee, oh*, and so on. It was tedious. After she pulled the mirror out of my throat and sat back in her chair, she was silent for a moment. She looked to the side. Then she looked at me directly, and said, "You've got a paralyzed vocal fold."

I explained that doctors had told me this was because of the tubes I'd had down my throat.

"It's not from any tubes," the specialist told me. "It's from having viral encephalitis. Sometimes it does that."

That was disconcerting. After a long pause I asked, "Will it get better? Is there anything we can do?"

"It may come back in a year or so," she told me. "If it doesn't, we can inject a filler to bulk up the paralyzed fold so it can close more effectively and then both vocal folds will work together to create a stronger voice. You'll sound normal for twelve to eighteen months."

"Will I have to go back in the hospital? I don't want to if I can avoid it."

"No, it's outpatient. You'd come in here, and we'd put you under general anesthesia and the whole thing would be over in about ninety minutes."

"General anesthesia?" My voice started getting louder. "The last time I went under *that,* I didn't wake up for two weeks."

"Well, then, let's wait to see if it comes back on its own."

I agreed, sighing with relief, and the doctor turned back to her computer, scrolling down my chart.

"We should get a CT scan," she said, "to make sure the nerves that invigorate your vocal folds are okay."

"But they did CT scans in the hospital of my entire body. Several times!"

"I don't see any for this specific area, but I'll look again and give you a call."

I was relieved when I could finally get out of this doctor's office. All of my recent medical appointments had been celebrations of my survival and recovery. This doctor had brought back the agonies of searching for the elusive source of my problems.

I was not going there again. I was fine. Everything was fine.

♦ ♦ ♦

A few days later, I was in the kitchen putting away groceries that had just been delivered when I got a call from the ear, nose, and throat specialist. She said that she had checked all of my records from last summer and there were no CTs of the internal laryngeal nerve. "That's what we need to look at," she said, "to make sure there's no injury and no tumors."

"Tumors?" I asked. "You mean cancer?"

"Well, yes."

I was stunned into silence.

"It would be very rare," the doctor said in a reassuring voice. "I'm sure everything is fine. We just want to be certain."

I promised to call the radiology department and rang off.

There was that word again: cancer. Feeling dizzy, I leaned over the counter and hung my head down. I was overcome with a sense of heaviness. I wanted to sink down to the floor.

They had spent weeks in the hospital looking for cancer, and they hadn't found anything. Meanwhile a ridiculous chickenpox virus encroached more and more into my brain. And now this doctor wanted to look for cancer!

"Again!" I said it aloud, desperation in my voice.

I made my way to the couch and sat staring out the window. The sky was a slate gray, and a dismal, depressing rain was falling.

"Very funny, God," I was still speaking aloud—and this time it was louder. I was almost shouting. "Wouldn't it be just a great cosmic joke if, after all those weeks of looking for cancer, they had missed it! This is just too much!"

I started throwing things around the room—books, papers, catalogs, whatever I could get my hands on. Fortunately, nothing was breakable.

I started moaning, "I just can't do this. I just can't do this. . ."

Chapter 30

LOOKING FOR CANCER AGAIN?

I didn't tell anyone about the CT scan. I figured I had already taken my family and friends through enough terror for now. I found that I was sinking into a spiral of anxiety, and so I decided I needed to go to the meditation center for a Friday evening satsang. I hadn't been back since that fateful day at the end of July when I'd become so sick.

It was a mild November evening, and the clouds had cleared enough that, walking from the parking lot, I could see a thin slice of the waning crescent moon along with a sprinkling of stars. When I entered the meditation center, a woman waiting for satsang to start, said, "Susan! Welcome back. It's so good to see you." She smiled and enfolded me in a warm hug.

It was Maggie, and it was good to see her, as well. "I haven't been here since Gurupurnima," I told her. "I started speaking in scrambled sentences, and Ann drove me to the hospital and then my 'great adventure' began." My stomach began to clench at the memory.

"Oh, my God," Maggie said. "I do remember seeing you with your coat on, sitting by the door. Why didn't you say something?"

"I guess I was afraid to talk."

Other people gave me warm-hearted greetings, telling me how well I looked.

In a few minutes, we entered the hall and sat listening to soft CD music while we waited for the satsang to begin. Candles flickered by photographs of the gurus, musicians prepared their instruments for the evening chant, and a stillness shimmered subtlety in the air.

Oh, how I had missed the peacefulness of this community.

After a half an hour of chanting we listened to a CD of the guru, giving instructions for meditation. Following her directions, I took deep breaths and inwardly said the mantra. Soon my mind became very quiet. I felt as if I were sitting outside on a beautiful beach, listening to the waves of the ocean and gazing at a luminescent silvery moon. At one point I opened my eyes and looked around the darkened room at all these meditating people. I felt that we were all connected at a deep level. It felt wonderful to be back.

Closing my eyes, I sunk deep into meditation and my worries melted away.

♦   ♦   ♦

"Do you want banana or vanilla flavored?" The radiology clinic receptionist was very direct, probably because she had to deal with so many reluctant patients. I looked at the two large bottles of barium that I would have to drink before the CT scan.

"I'll take one of each," I said, trying to be a cheerful Girl Scout.

I sat down in the waiting area with my bottles and straw, aware that other patients were watching me. I smiled at them, opened my book, and started drinking the chalky banana flavored barium.

Minutes later I walked into a bare room with a gurney-like bed and metal IV holder. I felt my breath catch.

It was like a hospital room. It was *too much* like a hospital room.

The radiology technician handed me a faded hospital gown to change into, but seeing my face, he changed his mind. "You can leave your clothes on," he said. "We just want to make sure your arm is free for the IV.

"Why do I have to have an IV?" I asked him. "What's in it?" My voice seemed to be growing louder with every word.

"Your doctor ordered an IV with contrast. So, the barium and the iodine-based fluid that's delivered through the IV, will highlight the laryngeal nerve."

"How will it feel?"

"You might feel like you're peeing your pants, but don't worry, you're not."

"Great," I said to myself as he walked away. My cheerful, good girl, rule-obeying demeanor was evaporating fast.

Soon, I was lying on an uncomfortable table with an IV poking out of my arm. The iodine drip burned my arm and chest. With my free hand, I pulled up a thin blanket I'd been given. I was still cold.

When was this going to be over? Never in a million years had I thought I'd be back getting another test to look for cancer. I was more scared now than I had been when they were looking for the source of my supposed brain cancer. I told myself everything would be fine if I would just repeat the mantra, but it felt like that was too hard. I just couldn't make myself do it!

After a long time trying to get comfortable and struggling to repeat the mantra, I got off the table with the help of the technician and walked into another room, where I lay on a metal table that moved through a donut-shaped machine while the scans were taken. The iodine fluid burned like the whiskey I used to drink, all the way down my body.

Later that day at home, I had cramps and diarrhea. Sitting on the toilet, I read about the possible side effects of barium. Diarrhea was one of them.

I felt anger flaming inside of my chest and stomach. Doctors should have to go through these horrible tests before they prescribe them.

A few days later, I got a call saying that the test results had come in and that everything looked normal.

"That is just great!" I said. "Oh my God, what a relief. And please tell Dr. C that I'll wait a while to see if my vocal fold regains its strength on its own."

Hanging up the phone, I felt so jubilant that I wanted to dance. I put on one of my favorites, a '60s song called "People Got to Be Free" by the Rascals. Backing up from my window so my neighbors wouldn't see me, I threw my arms above my head and moved my hips side to side and sang as loudly as I could with my one working vocal fold.

◆ ◆ ◆

A week later I sat drinking tea with a friend in a small Starbucks close to my home. I could hear the piercing sound of a blender grinding ice for Frappuccinos. The smell of coffee floated in the air, and a couple next to us talked quietly.

"I'm so confused," I said to Betty.

Her eyebrows came together with worry. "What do you mean?"

"I read on the internet that fifty percent of the people who have viral encephalitis *die,* which freaked me out completely. Then I realized that the article said that was only for people with the herpes virus, not varicella-zoster, which is what I probably had. And while fifty percent of those people don't die, about *a third* of them do. And for the ones who live, half have long-term complications—even if they were treated within five days."

"What kind of complications?"

"Oh, nothing much," I said, sarcasm lacing my voice. "Short-term memory loss, mobility issues, language and speech deficits, and on and on." I sighed. "I know I'm so fortunate that my only issue is a paralyzed vocal fold."

"Does it hurt?"

"At the end of the day it feels like I'm straining, and I can barely speak. But the doctor said my voice might come back in time on its own. Meanwhile, I'm going to chant as much as possible. Maybe that will help it regain strength."

Betty looked at me with concern. "I was so worried we'd lose you," she said. "But I didn't want you to come back halfway. I prayed that you either transition out of here—you know, move on—or come back and completely recover."

A shiver went down my spine. No one else had been quite so direct about this. But I was sure that others who had seen me curled up in a fetal position, mumbling or crying out something incoherent had quietly held the same opinion. I took in a deep, shaky breath. "I know. I am so lucky."

"If someone had asked me if I thought you and I would ever again be sitting here sharing our lives, like we are right now, I would have answered, 'Never in a million years.'"

"Yet here we are," I said.

"Yet here we are." She looked at me for a second. "Have you written the guru?"

"You mean to thank her?"

"Of course. The guru knew all about you being so sick. Your kids sent her flowers and asked for her help and protection."

I promised Betty I would do this, but I realized that I felt a little shy about writing to this great being. She had thousands of devoted followers and received many letters and cards asking for help.

Maybe I could just thank her and tell her how well I am.

When I got home, I looked through a collection of cards that I had purchased at my favorite gift shop. I needed to find the perfect card and write clear, humble, heartfelt words. Finally, I found one with a photograph of a beautiful yellow rose. I had a picture that depicted the goddess Shri Lakshmi holding a yellow rose to symbolize beauty.

It seemed like this was the perfect card for the guru, who is certainly beautiful. I wrote a simple explanation of my recovery and expressed my profound gratitude, and then I dropped this letter in the mail.

Chapter 31

BETTER THAN EVER

Soon it was the end of November. The trees were barren of their colorful leaves, and by 4:30 p.m. every afternoon the night fell like an impenetrable black curtain.

One drizzly gray morning, the phone played the first few measures of the Beach Boys' "Fun, Fun, Fun." It was Alena's ringtone. I picked it up with a smile.

"Hi, Sweetie."

"Hi, Mom. Guess what?"

"Nah, I'm terrible at that game."

"Come on, just do it."

"Okay. You got a big raise."

"That would be nice, but no."

"You and Zack eloped."

"No," she said, laughing. "Maybe later but not now."

"You're pregnant," I said.

"You got it. Zack and I are having a baby!"

My thoughts slowly drained out of me and seemed to float in a puddle at my feet.

"Mom?"

"I'm here. You haven't even known him that long. How far along are you?"

"About six weeks."

"Mom? Are you still there?"

"Yeah. How are you feeling about this?"

"Relieved, mostly. I thought I couldn't get pregnant. You know Ken and I were trying for a while, and nothing happened. So, I guess it wasn't me!"

"I guess not."

"Do you think you could be happy for me, Mom?" she asked, her voice growing soft.

"Oh, you know me. It takes me a while to process big news like this. It's just so sudden. Didn't you use birth control?"

"No," she said, sounding offended. "I didn't think I could get pregnant, like I just said."

Or perhaps she had wanted to get pregnant.

"So, Zack's taking Jude out of school and moving from Omaha to Lincoln, and we're all going to live together in a new apartment."

"I thought you just told Zack that you and Rowan needed to live by yourselves for the time being," I asked, my voice growing sharp.

"Well, not now with a baby coming."

We talked a little longer, and I tried to come up with more enthusiasm.

When we hung up, I called JoAnne and told her the news.

"A baby coming into the family? It's been so long," she said, sounding delighted.

Then I called Mary Lou with the news. She was equally enthusiastic.

After our conversations, I felt a little better but still wondered why Alena had to rush headlong into what would be a huge change in her life—and in Rowan's life as well. It seemed impulsive. I had no answer.

◆ ◆ ◆

A few days later I noticed a lot of hair in the sink and bathtub. I checked out my reflection in the mirror. Did my hair look thinner? I ran my fingers through my scalp and sighed. Well, it wasn't exactly thick!

My anxiety began to rise like a threatening thunderstorm. I went to my computer and emailed my primary doctor, asking her if there was any reason that I would be losing my hair. I knew that having lupus had caused some of my hair follicles to die and that they would never come back. So, I asked the doctor, "Could this be a lupus flare-up or did encephalitis kill my hair?"

I ran to the bathroom and looked at myself in the mirror again. I felt an urgent need to find out what was happening, so I dialed my rheumatologist's office and poured out my worries to one of her nurses.

The nurse responded with calm compassion. "I'm looking at your latest labs," she said, "and they're great, so it's not lupus."

"Well, that's good, I guess. Then what is it?"

"It could be from being in the hospital for so long. Your poor body was sick. It had anesthesia, surgery, and a lot of medication to deal with. Your hair is very sensitive, and it probably went into resting phase."

"A resting phase? Meaning it's not growing right now?"

"Right. But don't worry, it will grow back. I promise."

I thanked her and hung up. Despite her positive response, my anxiety sank to a kind of despair. I felt like going to bed for the rest of the day and reading a good mystery. Did I need to get a wig?

I didn't hide in bed, but like an insecure teenager, every time I passed a mirror, I stared at my head and wondered what was happening.

No one commented on my looks until a particularly pernicious dinner party. Some members of my extended family were celebrating their anniversary, and I was proud of myself for driving miles through rain and traffic to their party, which was in a restaurant in South Seattle. I wanted to regain a feeling of normalcy in my life, and it helped to go out for celebrations like this.

It was enjoyable catching up with family and honoring the special couple. During the goodbyes at the evening's end, a family member I hadn't seen for some time approached me. "It's been good seeing you," she told me. "I'm glad that you're feeling so well."

"Thank you so much. I'm better than ever."

As she gave me a hug, she whispered in my ear, "I can see that you're losing your hair."

Then she pushed me away, held me at arm's length and tittered.

I was embarrassed. "I know, it seems like. . . I mean, I guess I am."

I felt like I was apologizing to her. I said a hurried goodbye and went straight to my car to drive home.

Later, at a point when traffic was at a standstill, I thought about the exchange and burned with humiliation. I felt like I'd been pierced by an arrow. How could she give me a hug and then talk to me like that? Didn't she know how uncomfortable I was?

When I finally got home, I threw myself on my bed and cried. Alena was having a baby, moving in with Zack and his son. I would never have Alena and Rowan to myself again. And my hair was falling out! Was I going to be bald? What was I going to do? What could I possibly do?

◆　◆　◆

A few days later, Mary Lou and I went out for Indian food. Without telling her what my relative had said about my hair, I asked if she thought I should buy a wig.

She said, "You could get a wig, but I wouldn't worry about it."

Toward the end of the dinner, we had the waiter take a photo of us to celebrate our first time out since I'd been sick. When I saw the photo, I was shocked. My hair was thin, and my hairline was receding. I put it out of my mind and focused on enjoying my time with Mary Lou.

The next morning, I looked at the photo of Mary Lou and me again. I looked awful. I needed to get a wig.

I called my friend Mary K, who'd worn a very natural-looking wig when her hair fell out during her cancer treatments. She gave me the name of a wig shop in the Wallingford neighborhood, and in a few days, we went there together.

A friendly and soft-spoken woman sat me in front of a mirror. She had thick, wavy brown tresses that touched her shoulders. I wondered if it was her own hair.

"So, are you in treatment?" she asked.

"No, but I spent five weeks in the hospital being treated for viral encephalitis. For a while they thought it was cancer." I told her my medical story and finished with "So, after all of that, my hair started falling out."

"You've been through a lot," she said.

"You really have lost hair," Mary K said, looking down at the top of my head.

I cringed at that, but at least I was in the right place to deal with it. After a few minutes' discussion, I decided on a synthetic wig. It was cheaper and easier to take care of than one made of human hair.

It was fun trying on different wigs. Looking at myself in a long blondish upswept style, I laughed,

"Hey, I could wear this to a New Year's Eve party! Except I'm usually in bed around eight o'clock."

An hour later I walked out wearing a new light brown mid-length wig with gold and blonde highlights. The sun was shining brightly in a blue sky with white fluffy cumulus clouds drifting by. I felt a new confidence. A cute youngish man glanced at me and smiled. I grinned back, feeling great.

"Hey, that man just smiled at me," I told Mary K.

"Well, you look pretty good," she said, laughing.

◆　◆　◆

My new hairstyle inspired me to go out more. I had a lot of missed time with friends to make up for after my weeks in the hospital and rehab. I set up a date and met Jenny and Val at Starbucks. I was thrilled to be able to participate fully in life again and excited to see what they'd say about my "hair."

As Jenny and I nibbled on chocolate chip cookies, we listened to the happy hubbub of the crowd at our favorite Starbucks on Lake City Way. Val waved as she came in the door, went to the coffee bar and ordered something. Soon she set a giant mocha in front of me.

"Thank you, thank you," I said. "But after all you've done for me, I should be getting you one."

"You never got to drink the last one we bought, remember?"

"It was in the hospital," Jenny said, sitting down. "You were getting that transfusion so we couldn't take you to the sunroom and have coffee. And they wouldn't let you drink it anyway."

"So, here's to you, Suzy-Q," Jenny said, raising her cup.

We toasted and laughed and celebrated being together for a while. I asked them if they liked my new wig. They hadn't even noticed!

"It looks great and so completely natural that I thought it was your real hair," Val said.

We talked for a while about the dismay of losing my hair, the hurtful comment my relative had made, and Mary K's help in finding a new wig.

"You look better than ever," Jenny said.

Then our conversation turned more serious.

"I'm so glad things are back to normal," Jenny said, sighing. "I want you to know, Suzy-Q, that I had a little goodbye ceremony for you one night. That day Val texted from the hospital that your condition had turned grave. And when I got to your room you were curled up in a fetal position, eyes closed, moaning occasionally but otherwise. . . nothing."

Jenny paused and looked out the window. The sun was setting on another rainy day. Val was staring at the table, seemingly lost in thought. I felt as if an invisible hand squeezed my heart.

People had been saying goodbye to me. I had been that close to dying.

"When I went home, I had to write," Jenny continued. "So, I got my pen and opened my spiral notebook and wrote a letter to you. I wrote about how I would miss you and how I loved the grand times we had at Starbucks and celebrating our fabulous birthdays. I was preparing myself for the worst—a live body but not one that would really be you, the Susie Q we all know and love."

They were silent for a moment, lost in their recollections.

"I'm sorry, guys, for putting you through so much. There's so much I don't remember. I had no idea that things were that dire!"

"We're just glad you're back," Val said.

♦   ♦   ♦

The days flew by, and soon I was at a swamped Sea-Tac airport, checking in for my Christmas trip to Lincoln. I decided to get a wheelchair to the departure gate. Even though I no longer needed a walker or a cane, I knew I didn't have the strength to stand in line for an hour waiting to go through security.

When I got to the gate, I sat down in a tiny seat between two groups of people flying somewhere for Christmas.

I was so tired! Would I be able to handle the line at Starbucks to get a chai and a scone?

I stood up and looked. There were throngs of people in the corridors. I decided to forget about Starbucks. I didn't have the strength to stand that long. I went to the restroom instead. The stall for people in wheelchairs was full.

So, there would be no raised toilet seats for me. I was going to have to press my hands down on the toilet seat to get up. Why were the toilets so low?

After managing to go to the bathroom and boost myself up, I washed my hands for a long time. Looking at the mirror, I tried without much success to fluff my hair. This wasn't the wig, and my own hair was definitely thinning.

Oh well. Alena wouldn't notice. I had decided to leave my wig at home. It was hard to keep in place—and what if it had tilted sideways! I'd decided that it was too much to worry about.

Back at the gate people were beginning to line up for boarding. Standing at the end, I berated myself. *Why didn't I ask to board first? How am I going to get my carry-on bag up to the overhead bins?*

My shoulder and neck muscles tightened with tension. I focused on breathing and silently repeating the mantra. Intrusive thoughts persisted. *How the heck am I going to do this? I can barely get out of a chair, let alone a squishy plane seat. Will I have enough time to get to the connecting gate? Why am I flying through Denver? It is so big.*

With my thoughts beginning to spiral out of control, the line slowly advanced toward my first Christmas with Alena, Rowan, and their new family.

Chapter 32

WHY DID I GO?

I paused briefly and assessed the long flight of stairs ahead of me. "Is there an elevator?"

"Nope. This building is way too old," Zack said, smiling and shaking his head.

How the hell was I going to do this?

I'd arrived for Christmas at Alena and Zack's apartment in north Lincoln after twelve hours of traveling from Seattle. I'd used wheelchairs to get through security, but I still had to walk a long way between gates. I'd done great up until this moment. Now, I was worn out, and my legs felt shaky.

Zack asked me, "Are you okay?"

"I'm just a little tired," I answered, flushing with embarrassment.

"Okay, the apartment is right up these stairs and at the end of the hall."

He grabbed hold of my big duffel bag and began the trek.

I could do this. I'd just hold onto the railing and pull myself up. If I looked up ahead at the long flight, it would be daunting, so I focused on each step and silently repeated the mantra. As I marched upward, I noticed the brown-stained carpet under my feet and the musty smell in the air.

When we reached the second floor, I tried to slow my breath as I followed Zack down the hall.

"Here we are," he said, opening a door and ushering me into a spacious living and dining room. There was a sliding glass door, which opened onto a small balcony overlooking a long strip of lawn and large parking lot.

"Wow, nice big space," I said. "And look at this beautiful Christmas tree!"

"Yeah, the tree is all Alena. She picked it out at the tree farm."

"It reminds me of the kind of tree you see on the cover of *Ladies' Home Journal.*"

His eyebrows drew together in a puzzled expression, and I realized that he'd probably never even heard of the magazine.

Zack shifted topic. "Rowan and Jude have their bedrooms upstairs, so I'll take your bag up there."

Oh yeah, I'm sleeping in the same bed as Rowan, aren't I. That should be interesting. He doesn't move when he goes to sleep, but after a few hours, he's all over the bed."

"He's been having a hard time sleeping on his own since he's slept with Alena from birth. We've made a deal with him. He has to stay in his bed until 1:00 a.m., and then he can come downstairs and sleep with us."

I knew that would be difficult for everyone. "He's not easy to sleep with," I said from experience. "He moves around a lot."

"I know."

I wondered what they were going to do after the new baby came!

About a half an hour later, Alena and the boys arrived home from shopping. The boys said hi and ran upstairs. It was the first time Rowan had run off without at least giving me a hello hug.

I shrugged and turned my attention to Alena. She was dressed in a deep blue, silky blouse, which fell softly over her round belly. She looked radiant. Seeing me, she set the bags down and gave me a hug.

"Hi, Sweetie," I said. "It's so good to see you!" Patting her tummy, I asked, "Is there a baby in there?"

She laughed, and we talked for a few minutes about my flight.

"You are so beautiful," Zack said. He laughed as he hugged her, and he buried her in kisses.

Feeling uncomfortable, I headed upstairs to unpack a few things. Rowan and Jude screamed and ran past me.

"Quiet down, you two," Zack shouted.

This was going to be an interesting Christmas.

♦ ♦ ♦

Christmas Eve and morning came and went with the enticing aroma of cookies baked for Santa and the shrieks of excitement as presents were opened and enjoyed.

Soon after, Alena was back to work, and every morning I was awakened at seven to the sound of Jude's new, loud electronic toys, and Rowan pretending that he was a T-Rex.

Zack coped by reading the news and Facebook and, every once in a while, yelling at the kids to keep quiet. I sat nearby on the couch sipping my tea and trying to read my meditation website. Every so often, I'd try to engage Zack by asking a question about what he was reading. He'd give me a sweet smile and short answer with no openings for a conversation.

Late one long morning, I was lonely and bored. Rowan hardly seemed to notice me. Understandably, I'd been replaced by Jude. Neither of the boys wanted to play a game with me or create a story to act out. There had to be something I could do. An idea occurred to me.

"Hey kids," I yelled as they were running by me. "Stop for a minute."

"R-R-R-R-oar!" Rowan was shouting and arching his head and back.

"Rowan, can you be a *boy* for a minute and come here. Jude, you too. I have something interesting to ask you."

Zack watched us, eyebrows raised and a tiny smile on his lips.

In a couple of minutes, they ran over to me.

"How about," I asked, pausing for dramatic effect, "we go to a really fun, cool movie? *Star Wars*! It is supposed to be very exciting. Do you want to go?"

"I don't really like *Star Wars*," Rowan answered, looking away.

"I'm sure you'd like it, Rowan," Zack said.

"I've seen it, but I would go again," Jude said, jumping up and down.

"Rowan, the *Star Wars* movies are great adventures with fantastic special events. I've seen them since they first came out, and they're so much fun. You both could pick out your own treats too," I said.

He crossed his arms in front of his chest and shook his head emphatically. The answer was clearly no.

I was so disappointed. A bit later, I talked him into going to Barnes & Noble to use his gift card while Zack spent special time with Jude.

Right after we got to the store, Rowan chose a Lego set and was ready to leave.

"Hey, now that you've got your toy, what about a treat?" I asked, pointing to the coffee shop.

"No, I want to go home."

"You don't want anything? We always get a treat."

I so wanted him to say yes. This might be the only time he and I would have alone together.

"No, that's okay."

On the drive home, Rowan was very quiet.

The pewter sky and dirty leftover snow matched my bleak mood. Then I spotted a Dairy Queen approaching up ahead on my right.

"Look, there's our favorite place. Want to pull in and get Blizzards?"

Rowan sighed and mumbled another no.

I was bewildered. What had happened to the little boy who wanted to play with me all day and who loved treats?

As we came in the apartment, Zack looked up and said, "You're back already?"

"He wanted to come home," I said, shrugging my shoulders. I decided to try the movie again. I suggested that we all go, asking Zack if he had seen *Star Wars*.

"Yeah, let's go," Rowan said, finally sounding excited.

"I thought you didn't like *Star Wars*," Zack said.

Rowan sat down at Zack's feet and mumbled, "I'll go if Zack wants to."

"I've already seen it," Zack said.

At that, I gave up. "Okay," I said. "We'll go to a movie another time."

Jude watched Rowan as he spread the tiny pieces of his new set of blocks on the rug and tried reading the directions.

Zack read his phone.

I sat on the couch watching this new family so desperate to know where they all fit together, much like all the separate pieces of the Lego set Rowan was diligently trying to fit into a new whole.

◆　◆　◆

The days passed, one much like the other, with Rowan and Jude shooting at each other with their ray guns, Zack trying to be the stay-at-home dad, and me retreating to my room to meditate and nap. I looked forward to Alena coming home from work so we could visit, but her attention was divided by chores and spending time with Zack and the boys.

Soon, the last weekend before I was to leave arrived, and Alena and I were going to drop Rowan off at his dad's for the rest of the vacation. And I was going to finally have treasured alone time with my daughter.

As I sat in the living room reading my email and drinking English Breakfast tea, Zack hung up the phone and started singing,

"There's a storm coming to Omaha, and I don't have to go-o-o."

"What do you mean?" I asked.

"I was going to take Jude up to see my mom and stepdad's place for a Christmas celebration, but they're expecting a snowstorm, so I canceled. Now I get to stay here with you guys," he chortled.

"Oh" was all I could muster. Zack went to take a shower.

With the water running, he began singing a rock song from the '80s, and my stomach began to bubble with fury. I was finally going to have a chance to be with Alena—go somewhere with her that would be fun for the two of us—and now Zack was going to spoil it!

"Oh no," I said, covering my face with my hands. I slouched on the sofa, my arms crossed tightly against my chest.

Alena came into the room just then and, seeing me, said, "What's the matter, Mom?"

"I thought we were going to have today for just you and me, and now Zack has canceled his plans to see his mom. So, he and Jude are going to be here."

"What's wrong with that?" she said, furrowing her brow.

"Lena, I haven't had one single moment alone with you, and day after day all that I've done is sit on the couch and watch the kids run around. Zack doesn't even talk to me; he just sits and stares at his phone!"

"Mom, he's working," she said, sitting down on the footstool across from me.

"No, he's not. I've looked. He's on Facebook. And I sit and do nothing or go hide in my room. I swear I have been trying to figure out how to fly home early. But it's too expensive so I'm stuck!"

"Mom, this happens every time we see each other. Just like in Seattle when we didn't take you to the Space Needle. You just go crazy."

"Crazy. That's your go-to word to describe me whenever I don't behave like you want!" I could barely breathe.

This was not how I'd wanted to end this vacation. Why had I even come? This was just a disaster!

Chapter 33

COMING TOGETHER

Alena sat down on the rug and looked up at me. "Zack's a wonderful person," she said. "Can't you just be happy for me?"

"I know he is, Lena." My voice quieted. "But can you put yourself in my place for a moment? You asked me to come for Christmas. I didn't even think about the fact that I'd been out of rehab for only a few weeks and only recently able to get around without a walker. I really wanted to be here and spend time with you and Rowan in your sweet little apartment in south Lincoln. But then, suddenly, I'm in this big new place with Zack and Jude. And Rowan won't even play with me. . ."

"I want to play with you, Meemaw," Rowan said, looking up from a book. "It's just. . ." My six-year-old grandson looked at me with sadness in his eyes. I could tell he didn't know what to say.

I hadn't even realized he was there, looking at a book, and listening to his mom and grandma argue. I had been so caught in my own swamp of emotions that I'd ignored Rowan and his feelings.

I had forgotten about the huge transition this young boy had been through in just two short years. He'd been moved across the country, leaving his grandma and school friends behind, going to a place where the preschools were full and there was no Meemaw to take him on adventures. Within a year, his mom and dad were divorced.

Now, he was living in a brand-new household with Zack, Jude, and a new baby on the way.

I took a deep breath. "It's okay, Rowan," I said. "I just really miss the way things used to be."

Alena's eyes softened and her face filled with compassion.

"Okay," she said, pushing herself up. "We'll drop Rowan off at his dad's and then go to a movie."

"Really? Just the two of us?"

"Yes."

"What about Zack?"

"Zack and Jude will be fine. And Rowan can't wait to open all those Christmas presents at your dad's, right, Rowan?" she asked, smiling.

His face lit up. "Right!"

"Go get your stuff packed then."

Rowan ran upstairs to his bedroom.

Alena turned to me and added, "After the movie, we can get mani-peds." She leaned down and gave me a warm hug, and then she walked with conviction into her bedroom to set this up with Zack.

♦ ♦ ♦

I sat on a hard plastic chair in the crowded, stuffy Denver airport, waiting for my connecting flight to Seattle. Surreptitiously, I glanced at my hand, admiring my newly manicured and painted nails. I had chosen a deep rose color, and Alena had picked ruby red. We had so much fun that final day of my visit, talking and laughing. I finally got to see *Star Wars*. After the movie I discovered that Alena had already seen the movie with Zack, but she assured me it was fine for her to see it again.

I sighed with contentment. I was proud of myself for fulfilling my commitment to spend Christmas in Nebraska even though I'd made that promise before Alena had a baby on the way and she and Rowan were living in a reconfigured family.

I had known that I'd be pushing my body to travel so soon after being in the hospital and rehab, but I'd thought it would be fun and relaxing. It hadn't been that. Still, it had ended well.

"Good evening." This was from a loudspeaker. It was the agent at the kiosk speaking. I hoped she was going to tell us that it was time to board. There'd already been an hour delay. She did not say that. She said, "Flight 1592 will depart at 09:10 p.m. and will arrive in Seattle at 11:05 p.m. We are sorry for the inconvenience."

People grumbled and a few men went up and asked questions, speaking loudly enough for me to hear. I felt sorry for the customer service agent behind the counter; she looked exhausted with her wrinkled blue shirt and tangled brown hair.

I wondered how late we would be landing in Seattle. Would I end up getting sick from exhaustion? I tried to remember the time difference and flight time, but I was too tired to calculate. Instead, I slumped down in my chair and put my headphones on to listen to the mantra. I closed my eyes against the piercing glare of the fluorescent lights, but it was hard not to be bothered by my surroundings. Some-one nearby was eating a homemade sandwich that emitted the smell of bologna or some other mystery meat. And the plastic chair was uncomfortable. My butt hurt, and I was so tired.

When the mantra ended, I opened my eyes and saw an enchant-ing little girl with black glossy hair skip by me. She had pink head-phones on and was singing quietly to herself. She looked to be about five years old. I watched as her mom pulled out a plastic bag of al-monds from her purse and handed it to her daughter.

I wondered if Alena's baby would be a girl? If it was a boy, I'd have all grandsons. Of course, that would be okay. How would Ro-wan adjust to a new sister or brother? Out of everyone in his fledgling family, he was the one I was most worried about.

I opened my phone and brought up my latest photos. There were several from a beautiful snowy day. I'd woken up to bright light com-ing through the window and when I flung the curtains open, I saw gentle soft flakes drifting down. The world was covered in gorgeous white snow. Feeling like a kid, I'd opened my door and yelled, "It snowed!" Then we all got dressed, ran outside, and played. We had snowball fights, made snow angels, and attempted to make a snowman.

I looked at a photo of Rowan, Jude, and me standing together with our hats, gloves, and coats on, big smiles on our faces.

This was the most fun I had with the boys on this trip. It was the only time Rowan had actually played with me!

"Good evening. For passengers on United flight 1592, from Denver to Seattle-Tacoma Airport, there is now a new departure time. Flight 1592's new departure time is 10:10 p.m. and will land in Seattle at approximately five minutes after midnight. Again, we are sorry for the inconvenience."

A collective groan went out in our cramped, sweaty, smelly waiting room, and now at least ten people crowded around the gate impatiently demanding to know what was happening. I felt even sorrier for the harassed gate attendant, who was supposed to handle them all. She needed another person at that kiosk.

Trying to distract myself, I looked around for the pretty little girl. I stood up and stretched and then spotted her. She was curled up under a sweater, sound asleep in a little nest her parents had made for her on the floor next to the shiny window looking out toward the tarmac. Her mom and dad sat nearby looking at their phones.

Why did everyone have to look at their phones? What had happened to engaging in conversation? Why had Zack looked at his phone all day?

I then chided myself for being so judgmental. Zack hardly knew me. Perhaps he had felt uneasy or bored having to be the stay-at-home parent all week. Alena had told me when she called me in November that Zack and Rowan interacted really well, and I did remember seeing a sweet, funny interaction between them. It happened at a point when the two boys had been, surprisingly, standing still for a moment. They were in the living room looking down at the toys spread across the russet-colored rug. Zack walked by, took hold of Rowan's legs, and tipped him upside down, leaving his head and arms hanging. I started laughing, and so did Rowan.

"Zack! Let me do-w-w-wn. Let me down!" he shrieked. He was loving every moment of it.

"What's the matter, huh, huh, huh?" Zack was saying.

That little interchange was delightful. The problem was that Jude wanted in on it. He started saying, "Me too! Me too! Dad, hang me upside down."

When Zack finally turned Rowan right side up and placed him gently on the floor, Jude was right there with his, "Da-a-a-d! Me too!"

Zack, who was out of breath by then, could not just pick up another little boy. He told his son, "Jude, I told you before that I don't have to do everything with you that I do with Rowan."

Jude's face crumpled. With his body hunched over like he was an old man, he slouched over to the love seat and collapsed. The moment of lightness was gone. Rowan went upstairs to his bedroom with downcast eyes.

It was obvious that Zack was challenged by balancing his attention and energy between two active boys. Maybe that was why he had become withdrawn.

◆　◆　◆

I was brought back to my surroundings when a big man taking the seat next to mine inadvertently jostled me. These seats were so close!

Then another announcement came. This time we were told the delay would be several hours more. We wouldn't be arriving in Seattle until 5:00 a.m.

"This is ridiculous," I said aloud, and this time I got up to join the throng heading to the kiosk and two anxious-looking gate attendants. At least they'd gotten another agent to help.

I couldn't even get close to the front. People elbowed each other and shouted questions. A woman who looked furious marched away from the kiosk. Not wanting to be run over by her, I stepped aside. "What's going on?" I asked her.

"They said they can't find a pilot to fly the god damn plane from Seattle to Denver. So, our empty plane is just sitting in Seattle." And then she yelled to the ceiling, "I am never flying United again!"

They couldn't find a pilot? So, the plane was just sitting there at Sea-Tac? I slumped down on the nearest chair. Exhaustion weighed down on me like a pile of bricks.

Would I ever get home?

Chapter 34

THE LONG TRIP HOME

In desperation, I opened Facebook and posted that I was waiting for an elusive plane to take me home. In a few minutes many sympathetic messages came. I was feeling warmed by the support, when the speakers crackled. I peered at the gate agent, who had a neutral expression. I held my breath hoping we were about to board.

"Attention passengers on flight 1592 to Seattle. We are sorry to announce that, due to unforeseen events, the flight has been canceled."

"WHAT!" someone yelled.

"Please," the agent continued, "go to customer service to the left and down the concourse if you would like to be rescheduled. Again, we sincerely apologize."

People started running down the concourse, their carry-ons in tow.

I was not about to join that melee. I was too exhausted to compete. I put on my coat, pulled my heavy backpack onto my shoulders, and made my tired legs walk toward the customer service queue. It wasn't very long ago that my only way of getting myself from one place to another was with a wheelchair or a walker. Two months! And I'd been using a wheelchair for this trip, too. It was how I'd gotten from the check-in gates to boarding. Cold fingertips of fear tapped lightly in my chest. I needed to get home!

By the time I reached the line at customer service, there must have been a couple hundred people ahead of me. I began to complain to a woman standing ahead of me who had shadows of fatigue under her eyes.

"I can't stand in a line this long," I told her. "I have peripheral neuropathy in my feet and joint issues." I didn't bother mentioning my encephalitis adventure.

The weary lady I was speaking to was leaning against a man who had his arm protectively around her.

She said, "I can't stand in lines either. We're going to have to lose our place and go sit somewhere if this line doesn't move faster."

I felt sympathy for her, but also I was reassured to know there were others struggling too.

A young man who was walking by in that moment told us, "My friend and I just got new tickets down close to gate 13A. No line."

"Really," I said, surprised.

"Really. Right down there." He pointed behind him.

"I think I'm going to try it."

The couple gave me a doubtful bleary-eyed look as I left my place in line and walked away.

I trudged what must have been a mile until I finally got to the desk. There was no line. When I asked about new reservations for my canceled flight, the service agent seemed confused.

"We can't do that," he said. "You have to go down to gate…"

I interrupted him. "I know about the gate," I said. "I was just there." My voice got louder. "I cannot stand in a line that long." I went on to list my many maladies, again forgetting to mention the almost deadly encounter with viral encephalitis. Maybe it was too scary to say aloud. Maybe I didn't want to freak him out. What I did know is that I wanted to go home.

The agent called his supervisor, a woman who listened carefully to my story. She told me to sit down on a hard marble-looking bench next to the desk, and then she yelled at someone behind her, "She needs a wheelchair!"

I closed my eyes and took a deep breath, feeling a combination of embarrassment and relief. I had called a lot of attention to myself, but it seemed to be working.

A few minutes later, a voice said, "Okay, I think we have you taken care of."

I opened my eyes. It was the supervisor.

She told me, "We'll go back to the right place in a wheelchair and then get you a standby flight for tomorrow. We have a hotel for you to stay in and vouchers for meals. Do you want to stay in a hotel?"

"I. . . I think that would be great," I said, feeling humbled. "But I don't really need a wheelchair to wait in the line if it isn't for long."

"Are you sure?"

I had really pushed the disability thing. "I'm sure," I told her.

We walked in silence until we arrived at the gate. Now several hundred people were ahead of me. The tired couple I had left behind was still in line, about halfway to the desk. I took my place at the end of the line.

Ten minutes went by. My burning, tingling feet reminded me that I needed to take my medication for neuropathy. Was it time to take those pills? I had no idea what time it was in Nebraska, where I'd taken the last pill. . .how many hours ago? I was too tired to worry about it. My feet were telling me I needed to do something for them, so I found the bottle in my backpack and swallowed three pills dry. When I looked up, the supervisor was standing in front of me holding a ticket.

"Okay," she said, "I got you on standby for the first flight out to Seattle tomorrow morning at 9:00 a.m. You're number thirty-five in line."

"I've never flown standby before. What does that mean?"

"Thirty-four people are on standby ahead of you."

My eyes widened. "So, if I'm going to get on that plane, there have to be extra spaces for all thirty-five of us?"

"Yes," she said, "but it's the first flight out. Many of those standbys will get comfortable in their hotels and decide to sleep in, have a nice leisurely breakfast, and take a later flight."

"Okay." I sighed. "How do I get to the hotel?"

"Follow me."

As I walked past the line, I noticed several people glaring at me. I knew what they were thinking: *Who is she to get VIP treatment!*

I looked right back at them. I would trade with them. If they wanted the night in a hotel badly enough, they'd have to take my fifty-four years of lupus!

I never actually said it aloud, but my thoughts on this were very strong.

Soon, an electric cart shuttle took me and another grateful woman to separate taxis. I went then to an elegant hotel. My bedroom was huge, with a resplendent view of Denver. I took a shower and climbed into the king-size bed. It was 2:30 a.m., and I wanted to be back at the airport early. I did not want to be one of those people who decided not to make the flight. I set my alarm for 5:00.

◆ ◆ ◆

I couldn't go to sleep. I lay there thinking about my holiday.

One day, mid-morning, I'd been sitting on the couch having a cup of tea. I'd read everything I could on my email and the meditation website.

Zack, who was looking at his phone, handed it to me, saying, "What do you think of this?"

It was a photo of a ring with a gemstone that appeared at first to be blue. As I looked more closely at it, I thought it was almost white. It was lovely. The stone reminded me of billowy clouds on a spring day.

"What is this?" I asked him.

"It's Alena's engagement ring," he said, smiling.

It was a moonstone gem in a sterling silver setting with a sprinkling of diamonds on the side. It was absolutely beautiful, which I told him, and I also told him that Alena had been a little disappointed not to get an engagement ring for Christmas. "And here you had it planned all the time," I said.

I told him that I didn't know anything about moonstones, and he gave me a short lesson right then. Later, I couldn't remember what he'd said. The most important thing to me was that Alena loved Zack and that he obviously loved her. He was going to ask her to marry him.

Zack told me that he'd gotten airline tickets for Alena's best friend and her husband, so they could be there when he proposes on New Year's Eve. He was going to ask Alena to marry him somewhere outside, somewhere downtown by the Capitol.

In the midst of these happy thoughts, I drifted off to sleep. I was surprised when the alarm went off, and then I noticed that I felt pretty good for having had only a few hours of sleep.

◆　◆　◆

The airport was packed. I got a wheelchair to the gate and checked in there. I sat down and noticed that the little girl with dark shiny hair was awake.

"Did you guys stay here all night?" I asked her parents.

"Yes," her dad told me. "Didn't you?"

He was surprised when I told them I got a hotel, but they were number five in the lineup to board.

"I'm number thirty-five," I told him. "I don't know if I'll make it or not. Hey, I have a bunch of leftover food vouchers. Could you use them?"

He could, indeed. With a broad smile on his face, he went to get breakfast for his family.

I asked his daughter, "What's your name?"

"Mei," she said with a smile just like her dad's.

"That's a pretty name. Mine is Susan. Did you spend Christmas with your relatives?"

"Yes! We were in China, visiting my grandma."

"You're on your way back from China? Wow, that is a long way. What an adventure you've had."

"Yes, and I got all kinds of presents for Christmas. Wait, I'll show you."

She rummaged through her pink backpack and pulled out a box with a ballerina in it. She wound it up and a familiar tune played as the dancer turned in a circle. We passed the time congenially, and Mei told me about her trip. Her sweet company soothed the tender ache of longing I was feeling for Alena and Rowan.

After a while when the plane started to board, she left with her parents.

"I'll see you on the airplane, Susan," she said looking over her shoulder.

The group of remaining standbys began cheering whenever one of us got called to board. A fiftyish-looking man in a rumpled shirt had the last number, fifty-six.

"I'll never get on," he said with a sigh.

"Yes, you will," I told him—and I was sure he would.

He shook his head in despair.

Finally, my name was called. I walked into the cabin and found my seat. Mei spotted me and waved happily. When the plane was nearly full, number fifty-six boarded.

Many of us applauded calling out our congratulations.

"You made it," I said as he passed.

◆　◆　◆

I leaned back against the seat. I *had* made it. It had begun with two flights, then constant walking up and down the apartment stairs, little real rest, another flight, getting stuck in Denver, walking what seemed like miles in the terminal and then overnight with a modicum of sleep in a strange hotel. What a physical test! Like a ship in a storm that sees the sight of a welcoming shore, I was able to navigate through the tender exposed hearts of a new family and arrive safely with a better understanding of us all.

As the plane taxied down the runway, I thought of my next journey. In a month and a half, I was going to visit Lily. It would be wonderful to see her for the first time since my illness. But I felt uneasy about staying with her in the new house she'd rented with Matt.

Every time I spoke with her on the phone, she was upset about something that was going on with him. They'd had a big fight, he'd broken her phone, she felt forced to take refuge for the night on a friend's couch... There was always something that didn't seem right. Yet, she always went back to him. She'd said he had PTSD and that he just needed to get counseling. Nothing ever seemed to change, though.

I took a deep breath and repeated my mantra as the plane lifted into the sky. Looking down at Denver, I tried to relax. I was on my way home where I could rest and begin gathering my strength to take with me to see Lily.

I hoped and prayed I could somehow help.

Chapter 35

IT'S JUST IRAQ

The first day of my trip to Montana to see Lily was fun. She was proud of the new place she and Matt were renting, happy with the way she'd readied the guest bedroom for me with a new quilt and matching curtains. And the place was nicely put together. Lily and I went to see an international dance competition at a restored theater in downtown Missoula, and I took her out for a fancy dinner afterward. We laughed at how my wig kept tilting to the side, and we became teary-eyed at the thought of how close I'd come to permanent disability and even to death.

The next morning Lily went to work—she was a waitress at a restaurant downtown. I went for a walk that morning, and I meditated. Matt slept, and in the early afternoon he left on his Harley to pick up Lily after her shift.

A couple of hours later, they still hadn't come home, and I was worried. The three of us were supposed to be going out to dinner.

I heard the rumbling of a motorcycle and, looking out the front window, I was startled to see Matt and Lily drive by the house with Lily shouting at the top of her lungs.

What was going on?

A few minutes later, Matt burst through the front door, throwing Lily's leather satchel on the floor.

"Where's Lily?" I asked him.

He said, "She got off down the block. I guess she's pissed or something."

"Where did she go?"

"I think she's at that park. I don't know." He pushed by me then and went into the kitchen to get a beer.

I put on my coat and walked out to the middle of the street to see if I could spot her. Lily was walking toward me, and as she came closer, I could see that there was a look of despair on her face.

"What happened?" I asked her.

"Matt was supposed to pick me up after work," she said, "but he went to the VFW for a drink. For God knows how long, he drank shots of whiskey with his friends. He was blasted by the time he showed up to get me."

"Oh no," I said. I took her cold hands in mine, rubbing her fingers to warm them.

She looked around at the neighbors' houses. "Can we go find a place at the park and talk privately?"

◆ ◆ ◆

A few minutes later, we sat on the damp wood of a bench at a picnic table. Lily told me about her frightening ride home, clinging for dear life to Matt as he wove the Harley through traffic at heart-stopping speeds.

"He even passed cars on the bridge," she said. "I kept yelling at him to let me off, but he wouldn't stop!"

"That's just awful," I told her. "You could have been killed." In my mind's eye I could see Lily flying off the Harley and smacking into the concrete bridge.

"He was so drunk and angry. Did he go into the house?"

"Yes, and he threw your stuff on the floor."

"I can't believe he's acting like this in front of my mother." She put her head in her hands and sobbed.

Putting my arm around her I said, "It's okay, Sweetie. I'm just glad you got home."

"I bought new stuff for your room and everything. I just can't believe it. He gets so crazy when he drinks."

For a moment she was silent, wiping the tears from her face. She looked straight ahead and said, "Mom, if I moved out, would you help me out financially? I mean would you help pay the deposit on a new place? I'd pay you back."

The suggestion that she might leave Matt was thrilling to me. "Of course, I would help," I said. "And if you want to leave right now—I mean if you don't feel safe—you could stay with a friend for a bit while you look for an apartment, or even a room in a house."

Lily smiled. "I think my friends are all taxed out," she said. "I've spent so many nights on their couches."

"You have?" I asked. Why had I not known this?

"Yeah, Matt locks me out of the house when I come home late from work, so I call a friend."

"Oh, Lily. I can't believe he locks you out."

"Yep. I even have a backpack of overnight stuff and my sleeping bag in my car all the time. Just in case, you know."

The thought of this made my stomach roil with fear. Was there more? "Lily," I said, "does he ever threaten you? There are a lot of guns in your house."

"He's more likely to use a gun on himself."

I took her cold hands in mine again and looked at her straight in the eye. "Lily, listen. This is no way to live."

"I know," she said, her voice breaking. "If he'd just go to therapy at the Vet Center and get help. He keeps saying he will, but he puts it off."

"I, too, wish he would get help. But I'm *your* mom, and I want *you* to be safe. He could turn one of those guns on you. If you don't feel safe, and it's nighttime, get in the car and go to a friend's or drive to the airport and sleep in the parking lot. Then call me, and I will get a ticket for you to fly home."

"What about my job?"

As the sky began to darken, I tried to go through the many options she had for a different life. She was a bright, resourceful young woman. She could start over.

"You have my support, Lily. And your dad's. And Alena's! So many people love you."

"Thank you, Mom. That means so much to me." She shivered and said, "I'm freezing. Let's go home. Maybe Matt has calmed down by now."

When we got to the house, the garage door was open and loud rock music was pouring out. Matt was in the garage, singing at the top of his lungs. Despite my misgivings, Lily approached him and started speaking to him in a calming tone.

I went to my room and started putting my clothes and toiletries back into my suitcase. I had no intention of spending the night there. I'd get a hotel room, and Lily could come with me.

◆ ◆ ◆

A few minutes later, Lily and I were in her car, backing down the driveway. Matt was sitting on a chair in the garage, a glass of whiskey in his hand, listening to the raucous music.

"Wait," Lily told me.

"Let's just go," I said.

"No," she said, opening the passenger door. "I think I can fix this."

Lily spoke to Matt for a few minutes, and then he came to my side of the car. Reluctantly, I opened the window.

"I'm sorry," he said, twisting his body away from me. "You know, it's just Iraq. I can't help it."

What a bunch of bull that was. But I could see that he had severe PTSD. After a few moments of the two of us staring at each other, I relented and said, "Okay."

Eventually, Lily and I went out to dinner, just the two of us, and afterward I felt it was okay for both of us to spend the night at their house. I kept my suitcase packed and ready to go, just in case, and Lily promised she'd wake me if there was a problem.

I slept restlessly that night. The next morning, Lily took me to the airport, where we hugged and said a tearful goodbye. I hoped and prayed she'd call soon to tell me that she was ready to move out.

♦ ♦ ♦

Back at home after the trip to Montana, I reveled in the sweetness of my own peaceful life. I closed my eyes and tipped my face toward the sky. It felt so good to sit on my deck and breathe in the fresh air. The late February sun warmed my skin, and William was warm and heavy, sleeping on my lap.

I was relieved to be home. I wished I could help Lily, but she kept making excuses for Matt. She'd told me that Matt had apologized to her over and over for the scene he had caused the last day I was there. I felt discouraged and didn't know what to say.

I pushed the cat off my lap and went back into the living room, where I stood at the window watching crows fly past on their way to a roosting spot about seven miles east.

For some reason, I remembered the vision I'd had when I was waking from my semi-coma in the hospital. In that vision I'd seen Lily standing on stage in a crowd. Lily was shaking her fists and yelling.

Why had Lily been a part of that scene? Did this mean that I was supposed to help her get away from this destructive relationship she's been mired in? Is that part of the reason I got well?

♦ ♦ ♦

That night, I fell into a deep sleep. Then, at some point, I awoke standing in my living room with a thick darkness surrounding me.

It occurred to me that I was actually still asleep. I remembered that I had to find a light and turn it on. If the light didn't come on, it would mean that this was a dream and that I was still asleep.

In the darkness, I stumbled to the couch and felt for a lamp that I knew was on the end table. I turned the switch, and the light did not come on. Darkness reigned.

I knew then that I had to walk down the hall and get back to my bed. Suddenly, it wasn't as dark as it had been. There were tea lights lined up on the hallway floor—a string of tiny candles lighting my way.

Step-by-step, I followed the little lights down the hall to the doorway of my room. Instead of rushing to turn on the bedside lamp, I repeated the mantra.

My eyes opened. I raised my head and looked around my bedroom. The diffuse soft light of the moon streamed through my window, and I could hear the ocean-like sound of distant cars on I-5. I didn't bother turning on my lamp because I knew I was awake, truly awake. Not only because of the ambient light and noise but also because I could hear my phone playing the guru's sweet voice singing the mantra.

The mantra was really powerful! I had to remember that I could repeat the mantra to truly wake up. It seemed like a good idea to repeat the mantra a lot, whether I was asleep or awake.

Chapter 36

A Lot to Be Grateful For

The next morning in the bathroom, I leaned forward and looked at myself closely in the mirror. The circles under my eyes looked darker than usual. I wondered if my lucid dreams of being trapped in pitch blackness were affecting my health in some way. Was I really as tired as I looked? I didn't think so. Anyway, I could put extra concealer under my eyes.

I ran my fingers through my hair. It was growing back—and it was growing back curly! That was a shock. I said aloud, "I've never had curly hair in my life!"

I had no idea what to do with curly hair. I turned around with my mirror in hand and checked out the back of my head. No more big, round, ugly bald spots!

I could stop wearing my wig! People might notice the change—but so what! Why should I care what people thought?

With a wonderful sense of freedom, I left my sophisticated blonde wig on the mouth of the vase. I could wear it to a party some-day—though I haven't done that yet.

A little later I stood by my bed and pulled on my sweatpants and T-shirt. That was another felicitous change—I was getting strong enough not to have to sit while I got dressed.

Yet another change was that my voice was coming back. I sang a few rounds of scales, stretching out the final note for emphasis. My voice was much better! I wasn't froggy sounding anymore. The doctor had said that my vocal fold might not remain paralyzed forever. I was positive that the chanting I did every Sunday at the meditation center was helping.

In the beginning I'd been embarrassed at the way I sometimes croaked when I was singing. Fortunately, my fellow chanters never mentioned it, and they always welcomed me with smiles.

Later that afternoon, I called Alena to share some of my good news.

"Hi Mom," she said. "What's up?"

She sounded stressed. I said, "Sweetie, are you okay?"

"I just got home from work, and I'm getting dinner together."

I had forgotten that Nebraska was two hours later. Just then I heard her answer a question from one of the kids. Poor Alena was many months pregnant, on her feet working all day, and making dinner for a family. It made my news seem pretty small, but I told her anyway.

"I called to tell you that my hair's coming back. And it's curly! Isn't that just the coolest thing!"

"That's so great, Mom!" Alena sounded like she meant it.

"Not only that. My voice is coming back too. Listen." I started singing then in my best voice: "I'm looking over a four-leaf clover,"

She laughed. "You are absolutely right," she said. "I'm so happy for you!"

I could hear the pots and pans banging, so I said, "I'll let you go now. I know you're busy. But I just wanted to tell someone."

"Sorry, Mom. You know how it is around here after work: dinner, baths, reading, and then collapse into bed."

"I know. Okay, we'll talk soon."

"Maybe this weekend. Oh wait. Wait!" More clattering sounds came over the phone for a moment, and then, in an earnest voice, Alena said, "I've been thinking. Rowan is out of school at the end of May, and he's scheduled to be with me for a week. Jude will be with his mom then, and both Zack and I have to work. Do you want to come and stay?"

I hesitated. "I'm going to be coming in July after the baby is born, right?"

"Well, yeah, but this is the last time you'll get to be with Rowan by himself."

"Hmm."

"Zack," Alena yelled. "Zack! Can you get me the salt? In the cupboard above the sink. Yeah, right there. Thanks. Anyway— Mom? Are you there?"

"I'm here," I said. I was slumped down on the couch.

"Well? What do you think?"

I told her I was thinking about the expense of making two separate trips to Nebraska. I was also wondering whether I'd be strong enough to go up and down a million stairs—it seems like a million stairs—and run around with a seven-year-old ball of fire. And another worry cropped up, too.

"When I was there at Christmas, Rowan really didn't want to play with me. Do you think he'd be okay with me now?"

"Of course he will be."

It occurred to me that Rowan had been adjusting to his new family at Christmas—and that he would probably need my support. Anyway, it was clear that Alena needed my support. She was sincerely asking for it.

She said, "Why don't you think about it, Mumsie." I could hear the sound of tap water running in the background. She had so much going on right now.

"I don't need to think about it," I said. "I *do* really want to come."

We talked a few minutes more about the logistics of the trip and decided June was a good time.

After we hung up, I could still feel a tiny stream of fear trickling in my heart. What if Rowan was still upset and just wanted to sit in his room and play video games? Would Zack feel more comfortable with me staying this time? And what if I got stuck in Denver again? My health had been okay over Christmas, but there were no guarantees.

I told myself to shake off these fears. I just knew that God is with me, and I am with God. It's enough.

◆　◆　◆

The days sped by, and spring arrived in all its glory. It was the most wonderous season of renewal I could remember. Over the course of several mornings, I watched from my living room window as the blossoms on the magnolia tree plumped up and the tulip-shaped, fuchsia-colored flowers emerged and covered the branches of the tree. Beneath the magnolia, purple irises bloomed for the first time in many years along with huge, bubblegum-pink peonies. Deep within me was the knowledge that I could have missed this spring— I might not have been here for it.

One morning, standing on my deck and gazing at the beauty of the white, red, and yellow rhododendrons and azaleas that were in bloom all around me, I wondered why I didn't spend more time in my backyard. It was easy for me to access the backyard now, so that wasn't it.

It occurred to me that the backyard held bittersweet memories of playing there with Rowan. But I would be able to play with him again soon, I hoped.

Just the thought brought up my worries about traveling. I took another deep breath of the heavenly lilac-scented air and told myself that everything was going to be all right, that I would be just fine.

As it turned out, there was no reason for me to worry about the trip. It was perfect. The plane trips were easy, the three flights of stairs were surmountable, my energy was unfailing, and Alena and Zack were beyond gracious. They were both truly thankful I could be with Rowan while they worked. And best of all was my time with Rowan.

Rowan and I played outside in a park-like area I discovered on the backside of the apartment grounds. The spot had soft lush grass and tall cottonwood trees that created a cooling respite away from the glaring hot sun and the acrid smell of the parking lot's melting asphalt. While Rowan and I acted out imaginary characters, Zack's chihuahua ran around us in circles, ecstatic to be outside. It was such a happy time for all of us.

One day Rowan and I went with Alena to the obstetrician. By that time, we knew that the baby was a boy, and that his name was Sabastian. We all heard the magical sound of the baby's heartbeat, and we saw a round bump pressing up and moving across the inside of Alena's tummy. "Is that his head?" I asked.

The doctor smiled and said, "No. It's his bottom."

Rowan thought that was hilarious. He burst into laughter, and later he kept talking about how we'd seen the baby's butt.

We were creating lovely memories.

♦ ♦ ♦

Soon, summer arrived with its long days and stretched out twilights. One evening I walked to the grocery store, marveling at how much my strength had improved. As I carried the groceries upstairs, my cell phone began ringing. It was an 845 area code—which could be the ashram—so I answered it.

"Hello, may I speak to Susan," a sweet voice said.

"This is Susan."

"The guru received your letter about your vocal cord regaining strength after your illness and wanted to thank you."

I had almost forgotten about sending a thank you card to the guru—and now my guru was thanking *me*? I knew that without her grace and protection, I would never have healed so fully. I might not have healed at all!

The young woman continued talking, and as I listened to her, my entire being filled with love and gratitude. After I hung up, I danced and spun in circles around my living room, chanting God's name with the sweetest voice possible.

The guru is so compassionate and generous. Thank you, Lord, for this great master in my life.

♦ ♦ ♦

It was another cloudy day, and it was only the middle of July! I was going downstairs to the car—I had to get to a hair appointment—when Alena called.

"Mom," she said in a casual voice, "am I allergic to penicillin or is that Lily?"

"What?" I asked, confused.

"I'm checking into the hospital, and they want to know. It seems like one of us is allergic to sulfa drugs. Is it Lily or me?

"It's Lily, but why are you checking into the hospital?"

"Apparently, I'm in labor."

"Oh. My. God. When did it start?"

"I think about three hours ago, while I was at work. I had to go to a meeting, so I ignored the contractions—even though they kept getting more intense. It took so long for Rowan to be born that I decided not to worry."

"You stayed at the meeting?" I asked, my voice getting a bit shrill.

"Yeah," she answered, laughing a little. "When I saw my obstetrician, she said that not only was this baby on his way, but I was five centimeters dilated."

"Wow! But you don't sound like you're in labor. I mean, you're not panting or anything."

"I'm not in a lot of pain, and it is past my due date." It sounded like she cupped her hand over the mouthpiece while she answered someone else's question. Then she told me, "I'd better go. They want to check me in."

"Is Zack coming?"

"Of course! He's on his way."

"Okay, Sweetie. It feels weird that I'm not there for the birth like I was with Rowan."

"I know. Gotta go, Mom."

"Okay. Yay, a baby is on its way!"

As I drove to the hair salon, I thought about this exciting news. Who would have thought that a year ago Alena would be having a baby boy, and that they would name him Sebastian? Had Alena even met Zack a year ago? I didn't know. I'd been in the hospital then, in a semi-coma.

When I checked in with my hairdresser, I asked her if this cut was going to take away all of my curls.

"I think so," she said.

I didn't like that. I wanted to keep my curls. Surely, the hairdresser understood how great it was for me to have thick and curly hair—she had been the first person to tell me I had bald spots all over the back of my head.

Had that been the first symptom of viral encephalitis? No. I suddenly understood that the first sign was when I was startled out of meditation by the touch of something icy.

The thought made me shiver.

"You cold?" the hairdresser asked me.

"A little."

"I'll get you some warm towels from the dryer."

She was so nice. I should just tell her not to cut my hair short.

She smiled as she wrapped the warm towels around me, and I was touched by this simple act of kindness. I decided to tell her that a new being was on the way.

"Guess what!" I told them. "My daughter is in labor right now!"

"Your daughter's having a baby?"

"Yes, isn't that just wonderful? What about you? Any babies on the way?" I knew that she'd been trying to get pregnant.

"Not yet, but soon. I just know."

A little while later, I was reading my book as the stinging hair color seeped into my scalp. I heard my phone chime; I'd gotten a new message. I opened the phone and found a picture of a tiny baby, fist in his mouth and wide bright eyes.

"The baby is already here," I shouted. "Look at this photo. My daughter had a baby!"

People gathered around, smiling and saying how aware my new grandson appeared to be.

It was true. Sabastian looked like he was excited about life and ready for anything.

I texted my congratulations and my surprise at how quickly Sebastian had come. Zack texted back that their son had been delivered only forty-five minutes after Alena was checked into her room.

While I was forwarding the news and Sebastian's photo to Lily, Earl and Reva, Mary Lou, and JoAnne, I couldn't stop smiling.

What an amazing journey this year had been. Today was July 19. In twelve days, it would be exactly one year since I'd begun the incredible, transforming journey of my near-death rendezvous with viral encephalitis.

What a miracle that I was here at this moment, alive and healthy.

Soon, I would be holding my new grandson in my arms. Maybe I'd sing, "I'm Looking Over a Four-Leaf Clover" while I rocked him to sleep. I couldn't wait to look into those beautiful, shining eyes.

Joy filled my heart and gently streamed throughout my body. I took a deep, grounding breath. I was grateful to be alive.

STICKING AROUND

I t's been ten years since I navigated the perilous and transformative year that began in the summer of 2015. A lot that's wonderful has happened in my life in the intervening years.

In the fall of 2017, Alena and Zack married and moved their newly blended family into a beautiful classic brick house across the street from an elementary school in Lincoln, Nebraska. My secret dream was to live down the street from them, but at the time this didn't seem possible.

The next spring, I received a midnight call from Lily. She and Matt had just had a terrible and dramatic fight. Eventually the police had come, and he had been told to find another place to stay "for a while." For the next several hours Lily talked to me about how her relationship with Matt had deteriorated—what the nature of their arguments had started to be and how physically abusive he had become. He had broken her nose more than once, and he'd destroyed her phone a couple of times to keep her from taking photographs of her injuries. He had continued his threat to commit "suicide by cop" if she called the police. Thankfully, the nature of this fight was so horrible, the police were called.

The next day, Alena flew to her sister's side and—with the help of their nieces—they packed up Lily's belongings and drove her and her puppy to Seattle. Lily lived with me for a month, and then she moved in with a friend who lived in a town on the western slope of the Rockies in Montana. Over time, Lily rented her own place, found a job, started editing a book she'd been writing for years, and began to establish a new circle of friends.

♦ ♦ ♦

For several years, I continued living in the same house in Seattle. My beloved feline companion, William, went to a hospice for cats and then passed on—complications of cancer. I missed him, of course, and my house itself became increasingly difficult to maintain properly. There was always something that needed repair, and some of it was pricey—I had to take out a loan for a new roof. To bring in some extra money, I had the master bedroom and bath remodeled so I could rent them out to short-term guests. My plan was to sleep in the much smaller guest room and to use the main bathroom.

Late one evening in 2019, when the photos of my prospective rental space had been approved and the contracts had been written, the management company I was working with told me to wait twenty-four hours before I posted my advertisement online. The way they put it was, "Let's make sure that this is what you really want to do." What great advice that turned out to be!

The next morning, I got a call from Alena, who asked me if I could possibly move to Nebraska to be close to their family. She said, "I was telling Zack that I have no one living here who's from my side of the family and can love the kids as much as I do. Sebastian is at home most of the time, and he's so active that he needs to be playing outside. I'd love to have you spend the kind of time with him that you used to spend with Rowan."

The upshot was this: "Zack and I would love it if you could move here. And so would Rowan and Jude! And, of course, we'd be able to be there for you whenever you needed us."

There was no question about my answer was. I said "Yes!"

This was the end of October 2019. I was ready to hire a moving company, put my house on the market "as is," and be in Lincoln for Christmas. My realtor talked me out of so precipitous an action—I certainly would have lost money on the sale. So, in February 2020, with my house being newly painted, spruced up, and almost ready to go on the market, Alena flew in, and the two of us drove to Nebraska in a fully packed car. We arrived in Lincoln on leap day, February 29, 2020. (I take heart in the timing, as tradition has it that anything begun on this day is destined for success.)

In Lincoln, I lived in an Airbnb for a while and then bought a beautiful three-story, hundred-year-old Craftsman house in a neighborhood with cobblestone streets and lots of children. My plan was to organize block parties, exchange treats, and, for the holidays, frost Christmas cookies with the neighborhood kids, like I'd done in Seattle. This, alas, was not meant to be. Although everyone was friendly to *me*, some of the neighbors did not like each other, so block parties were not a possibility. Also, the traffic on the east side of my house echoed into every room, even after I put in new double-paned windows.

After I'd been there a year and a half, the stairs became a painful problem to my aging joints. One day when everyone was at work, I jogged up the outdoor stairs like an ebullient teenager—except that I didn't lift my foot high enough on one step and fell face down onto the cement steps. I was stunned and hurt. There was no one around to help, and my phone was in the house. I sat for a while, looking at the deserted streets and feeling forlorn. I was in excruciating pain. With sheer will and determination, I managed to make it inside and to call Alena. I was diagnosed with a cracked sternum and a torn rotator cuff. With physical therapy, I fully recovered, but something had shifted inside me. I no longer felt safe in my own home. What if I'd fallen down the stairs inside the house and couldn't get up! So, the following spring, 2022, I sold my house and bought a two-bedroom, one-level condo in a quiet retirement community. I missed living in a house, but now when I wake up in the middle of the night, I sense that there are people all around me—people who care and are willing to help if need be.

In 2024, just as this book was being prepared for publication, Alena and Zack decided to divorce—and my presence nearby became an even greater support for my youngest daughter and her two sons. I treasure the time that I am able to spend with Rowan and Sebastian. I am finding that it is such a privilege to be a part of their young lives, watching them grow and getting to hear their unique and mutable perspectives.

I miss many of my old Seattle friends and neighbors and, of course, my siblings and their spouses, all of whom I had to leave behind when I moved from the beautiful Pacific Northwest. However, living close to Alena and the boys has satisfied an inchoate loneliness and longing for family. And I make it a point to visit "home"—my beloved Seattle—often.

◆　◆　◆

Because I moved to Nebraska at the beginning of the pandemic—when people around the country, and even around the world, were shutting down schools, churches, and many businesses—I had a lot of alone time in which to ponder what the experience of my being so sick had actually meant. I believe now that the "icy touch" that initially startled me during meditation was from some departed ancestor, a soul making the journey back from the realm beyond life, to warn me to take care of myself.

I had neglected having blood tests that were supposed to be an every-eight-week routine for me. I needed to check my blood count because the medication I took to counteract lupus tends to suppress the white blood cells. Those blood tests would have revealed that my white blood count was dangerously low. If my doctor and I had seen that, then perhaps the whole chain of events that almost ended my life could have been avoided. I haven't had this "icy touch" experience since, but if it—or anything like it—ever comes up again, I will immediately pay attention to it.

The reoccurring dreams that so terrified me have ceased. If I wake up at night and there seems to be no light or sound, my first instinct is to reach over to my table lamp and turn the on the light. If the light doesn't come on, I know that I'm dreaming. Occasionally when this happens, I will decide to "go flying." My conscious awareness—what I think of as "me"—then zooms out the window, flies into the night, and goes exploring. Sometimes I fly straight up and joyfully sing whatever comes to mind; other times I simply float in the wind. Or I might remain in bed, feeling slightly annoyed and then relieved when I wake up, hear the sound of the mantra playing, and see the ambient light in my room. I still wonder if the frightening nature of my dreams shortly after I got home from the hospital was due to a part of me knowing that, for at least some of my time during my illness, I was unable to come back to being fully awake. Perhaps my consciousness was floating around, trying to "get back to my body," struggling to become completely aware.

♦ ♦ ♦

And what brought me back? Why did I get to live, anyway? Why am I now able to walk, to speak, to think? The simplest answer for me is that I had more to do. The vision in the dark theater, where I felt as if I were about to disintegrate into oblivion, was stopped when I saw Lily on the stage and remembered my identity as a mom. My love for her brought me back. But why was she shaking her fist and yelling? I think it's because she was in an abusive relationship and needed my help. What she did *not* need, I found, was for me to solve her problems and make everything easier for her. When I tried to "help" my daughter in this way, it only undercut her self-confidence; it only got in her way. I had to communicate my belief in her as an intelligent, capable adult. It took some time for both of us to get it right, but now Lily has established a happy and abundant life, and our relationship is better than ever.

I look back at the time of my illness, and I can see that I was given so much support and love. I will never be able to fully repay Mary Lou, Val, Jenny, Mary K, Barb, my beautiful family members, the meditation community, and the expert care I received from my doctors, nurses, and technicians.

At my latest birthday celebration, I had just turned seventy-six and, as the tradition in my family goes, each family member expressed why they were grateful for my presence in their life. Everyone had something sweet and lovely to say. Rowan's share, however, brought tears to my eyes.

Now fourteen, Rowan said, "Meemaw, I was thinking about how you've *always* been in my life. When I was little, you used to come all the way to Olympia to see me, didn't you? I realize that now, you're still here with me in my life." I looked into his bright blue eyes, and I saw that our beautiful connection was not only present, but it had deepened. My heart brimmed with love.

Later, I thought about the meditation I had right before his family moved from Seattle to Lincoln. In this dream-vision, Rowan had asked me, "Will you be there for me?"

So far, I have been. And I plan to stick around for a long time.

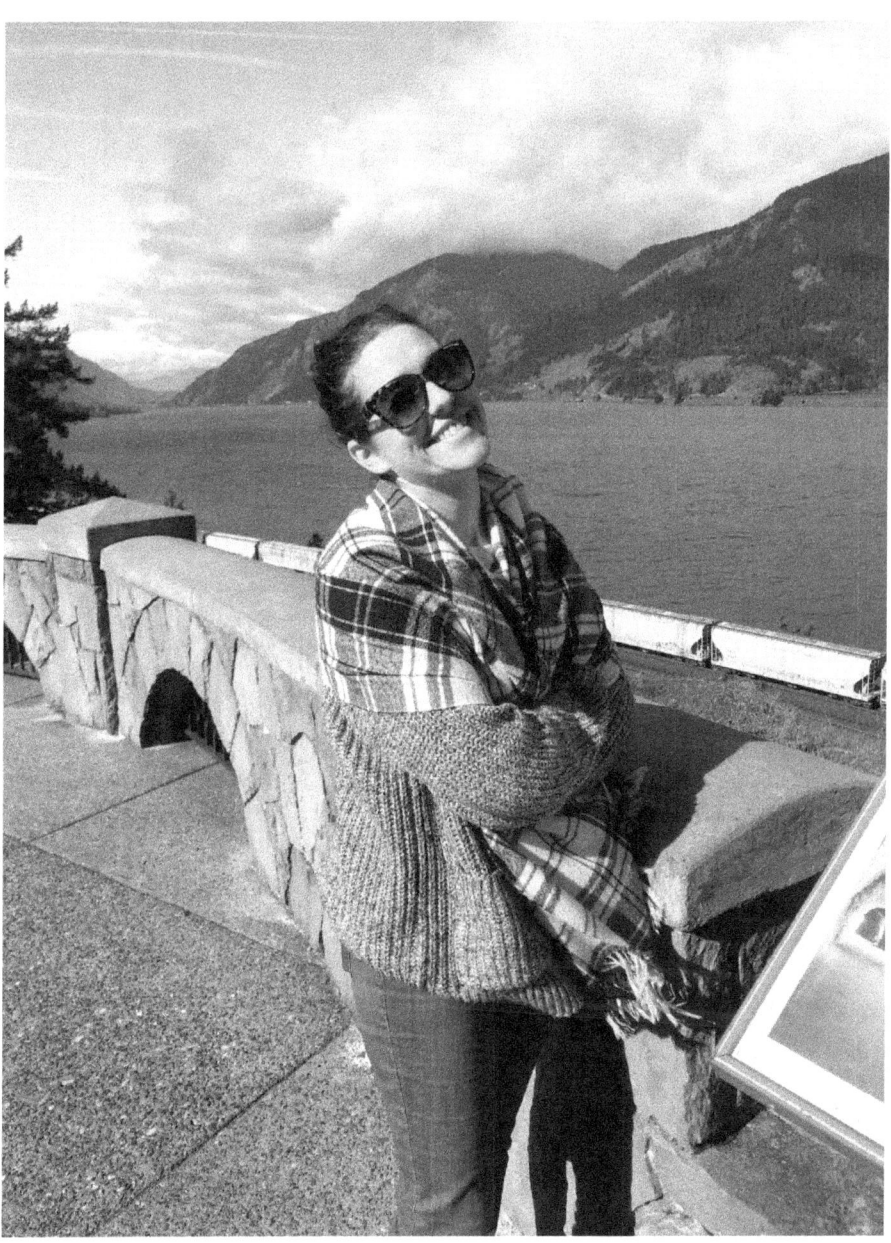

Alena enjoying Hood River during the first day of my move to Nebraska. We arrived in Lincoln three days later on February 29, 2020.

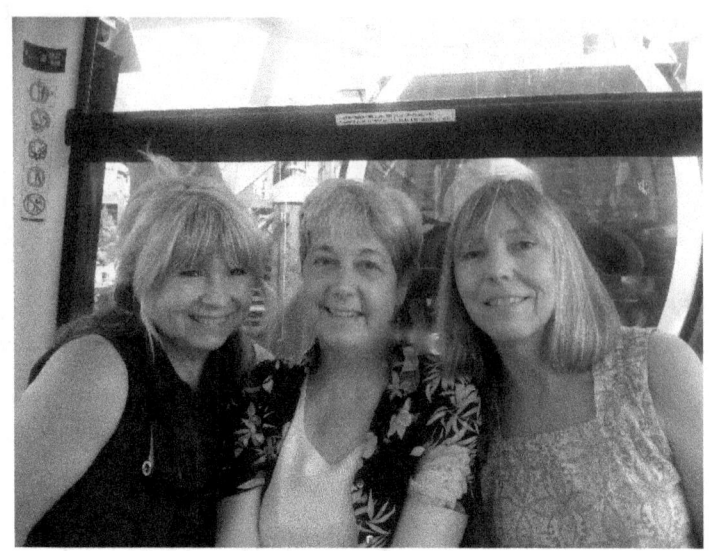

On the Ferris wheel overlooking Seattle with Val and
Jenny celebrating my sixty-fifth birthday.

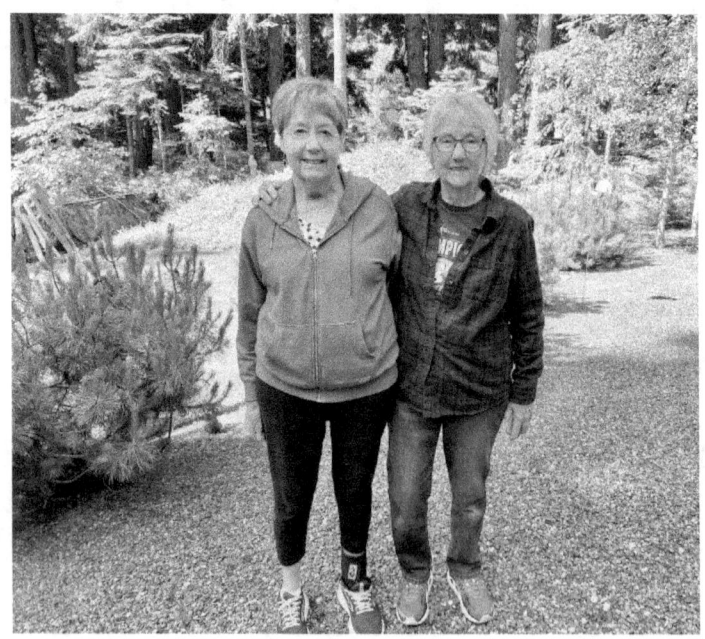

Childhood friend Barb and I at her home in Eastern Washington.
I visit her every summer and enjoy our adventures together.

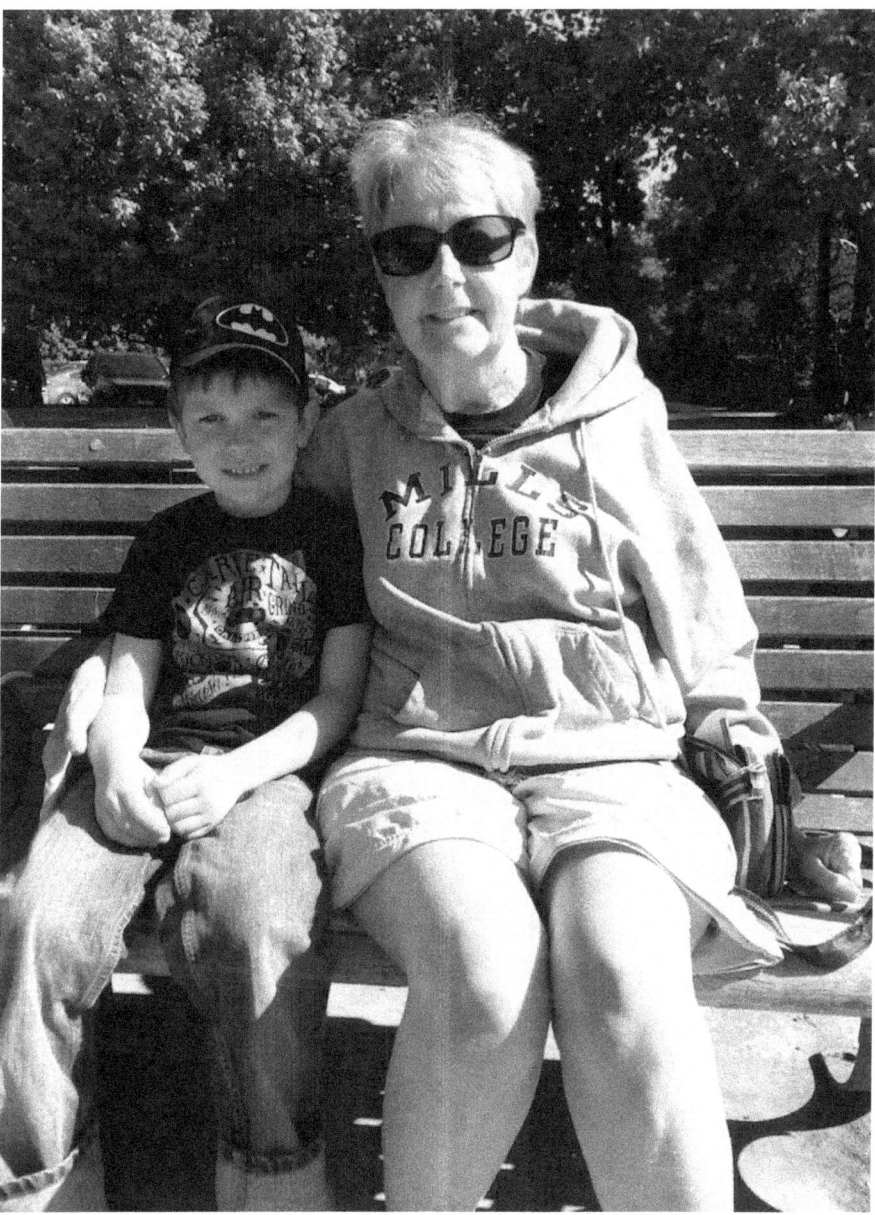

September 2015 with Rowan and I at Green Lake, our favorite place in the world. He cheered me on as I trudged determinedly with my walker all the way from the parking lot to the bench.

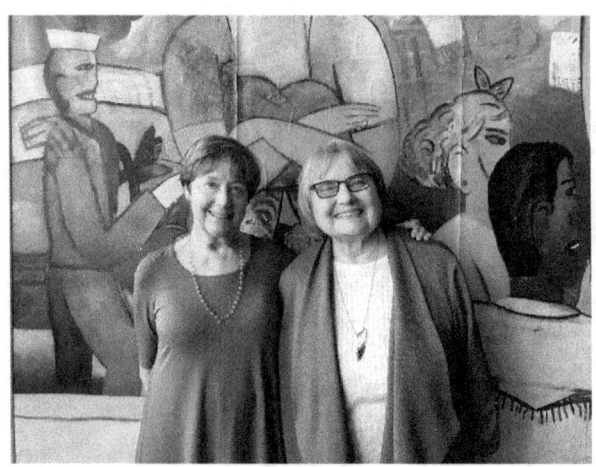

Mother's Day with Mary Lou at A Midsummer Night Dream ballet
in Seattle. We often spent this day together when our children lived out of state.

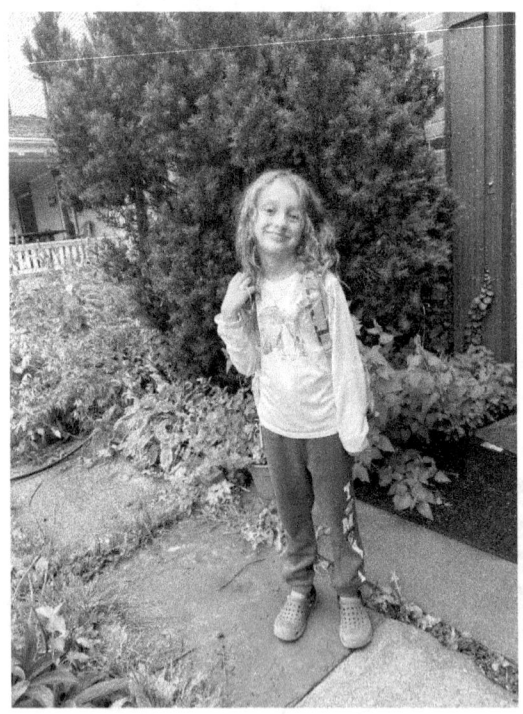

Sebastian on the first day of school 2024.
He was eight years old and starting the second grade.

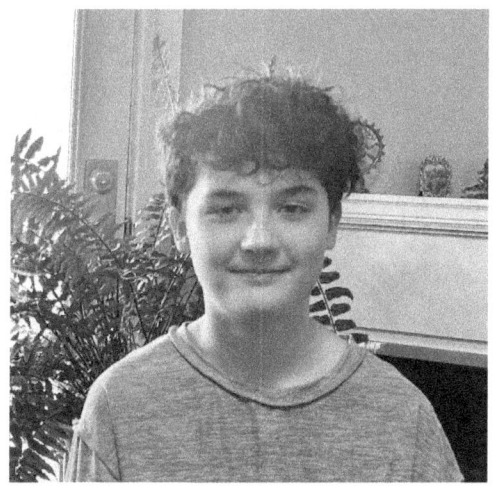

At age fifteen, Jude has grown into a handsome young man!

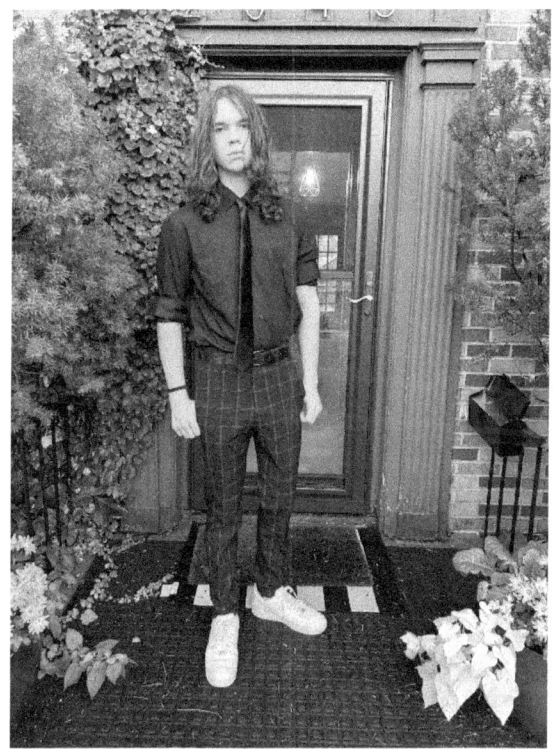

A very debonair Rowan posing in front of his home.

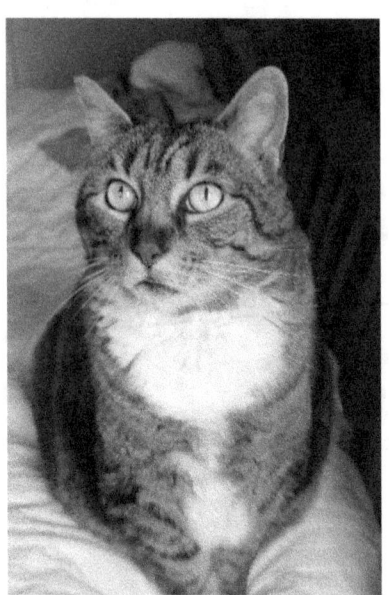

William the cat lived a long and happy retirement with me.

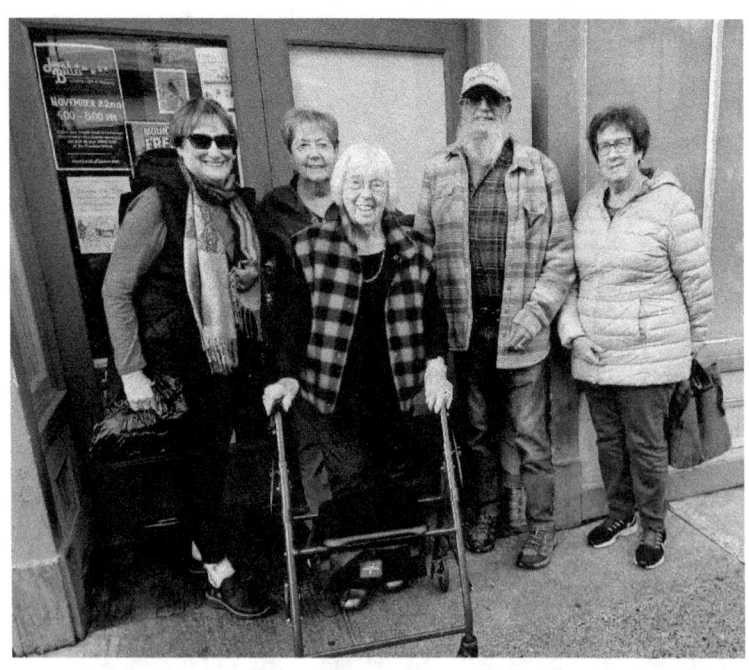

A sibling reunion for the first time in many years in October 2024. From left to right Nadine, Me, Earl, JoAnne, and (sis-in-law) Reva in the front.

ACKNOWLEDGMENTS

I wrote this book out of gratitude for my family, friends, fellow meditators, and members of the medical community—all of whom offered me support that, as it turned out, was absolutely necessary to bring me back to a state of health and well-being.

Most importantly, I am grateful for the guidance and protection I received from my spiritual teacher and from her path. The power of meditation, prayer, and the recitation of sacred texts that I did myself and that friends and family performed on my behalf greatly comforted me and, I am certain, helped to heal me.

I have a deep appreciation for my daughters, Lily Bruzas and Alena Bruzas; for my sisters, JoAnne Imholt and Nadine Smith-Cook; for my brother and sister-in-law, who are identified in these pages as Earl and Reva; and for my niece, Anita Coulson. I am indebted to my dear friends, Mary Lou Finley, Val Morris-Lent, Jenny Ross, Barb Pinney, Ann Shepherd, Katherine Dobson, and Mary K McCoy. These generous souls were a life-support to me in my illness, and several of them helped me in the writing of this book by allowing me to include their words to describe the difficult, and sometimes brutal, time I had in the hospital. Although I had little or no awareness during some periods of my treatment, these sweet souls let me convey my story through their voices.

I also want to thank the many members of my meditation and professional community who visited me at the hospital or the rehab center, sent flowers and cards, and said prayers. Thank you to (the now late) Beth Burrows for her daily get-well cards and visits, Mary Anderson, Lisa Barton, Juanita Rashid, Johnny and (the late) Yvonne Palka, Bonnie Bledsoe, Erin and Dan Johnson, and Pam Smith. I know there are others who came for visits while I was sleeping or when my poor brain wasn't registering. Even so, their presence was felt by me and often made it easier for my family. And what would I have done without my

Seattle neighbor, Diane Simpson, who took care of my cat, William, throughout my stay in the hospital!

I am also very grateful to my doctors—Dr. Paul Thottingal and two other specialists who are identified in these pages as Dr. P. and Dr. H. All of these medical professionals were instrumental in guiding my recovery and in helping me to understand why I became so ill. At a later appointment, when I told Dr. P. that I was writing a memoir, he enthusiastically brought out my brain MRIs. Enough time had passed for me to view them with detachment, and I was fascinated to go over them with him. He also had a staff member copy the MRIs so that I could keep them. Dr. H, in particular, spent hours helping me with the accuracy of my interpretation of my medical records—and has stayed in touch through cards and texts. I am also beholden to the staff and specialists at Virginia Mason Medical Center and the Post-Acute Rehab of the Foss Home and Village in Seattle.

♦ ♦ ♦

My initial foray into finding expression for this extraordinary life experience was in three writing classes I took at North Seattle Community College. I will be forever grateful to the teacher of these classes, Joanne Horn, for her encouragement and inspiration and for the writing skills she taught me. She always wrote, "keep on writing" at the end of my papers, and if I can track her down, I will send her this book to show her that I did!

Several of the members of these classes created an ongoing writing group that I joined, and this, too, was vital to my process of creating this book. I loved meeting every week at our various homes around the city, and I enjoyed our discussions of each person's writing. Members of this group were Barb Reid, Gary Lester, Rose Morris, Pete Dudley, Jean Swenson, Donna Parker, Nora McBride, the late Bill Crossman, and—last but by no means least—Tamara Pinkhas. Tamara later served as a manuscript reviewer—what's often called a beta reader—and her careful edits and suggestions were a tremendous support to me. This book would probably still be languishing on my old computer if it hadn't been for Tamara's taking the time to read each chapter and send it back to me—three times in all. My other esteemed beta readers were Bonnie Bledsoe, Linda Russell, and Michele Coleman.

♦ ♦ ♦

I want to offer special thanks to my editor, Margaret Bendet, for her graciousness and her many skills. She is a whiz and a true wordsmith!

ABOUT THE AUTHOR

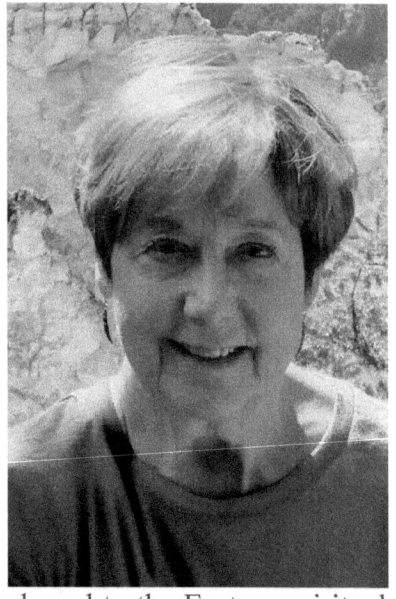

Susan Bruzas, a retired speech and language pathologist, decided to write about the compelling year she spent dealing with a "mystery" illness that none of her doctors expected her to survive. She now lives quite happily in Lincoln, Nebraska, and takes delight in spending time with her grandchildren, traveling overseas, and returning to the Pacific Northwest—where she resided for many years and where her medical drama took place. Susan credits her cure not only to her doctors but also to her daughters and many supportive friends and to the Eastern spiritual path she has followed for decades. She meditates daily.

www.ingramcontent.com/pod-product-compliance
Lightning Source LLC
Chambersburg PA
CBHW071718120626
46550CB00001B/288